Learnir
Hunti

of related interest

Alzheimer
A Journey Together
Federica Caracciolo
Foreword by Luisa Bartorelli
ISBN 978 1 84310 408 7

The Man who Lost his Language
A Case of Aphasia: Revised Edition
Sheila Hale
ISBN 978 1 84310 564 0

Stroke Survivor
A Personal Guide to Recovery
Andy McCann
Forewords by Robin Sieger and The Stroke Association
ISBN 978 1 84310 410 0

Dancing with Dementia
My Story of Living Positively with Dementia
Christine Bryden
ISBN 978 1 84310 332 5

Advance Directives in Mental Health
Theory, Practice and Ethics
Jacqueline Atkinson
ISBN 978 1 84310 483 4

Career Success of Disabled High-flyers
Sonali Shah
ISBN 978 1 84310 208 3

Law, Rights and Disability
Edited by Jeremy Cooper
ISBN 978 1 85302 836 6

Reconceptualising Work with 'Carers'
New Directions for Policy and Practice
Edited by Kirsten Stalker
ISBN 978 1 84310 118 5

Quality of Life and Disability
An Approach for Community Practitioners
Ivan Brown and Roy I. Brown
Foreword by Ann Turnbull
ISBN 978 1 84310 005 8

Learning To Live With Huntington's Disease

One Family's Story

Sandy Sulaiman

Jessica Kingsley Publishers
London and Philadelphia

First published in 2007
by Jessica Kingsley Publishers
116 Pentonville Road
London N1 9JB, UK
and
400 Market Street, Suite 400
Philadelphia, PA 19106, USA

www.jkp.com

Library of Congress Cataloging in Publication Data

Sulaiman, Sandy, 1959-
  Learning to live with Huntington's disease : one family's story / Sandy Sulaiman.
    p. cm.
  ISBN-13: 978-1-84310-487-2 (pb)
  ISBN-10: 1-84310-487-3 (pb)
    1. Sulaiman, Sandy, 1959---Health. 2. Huntington's chorea--Biography. 3. Huntington's chorea--Patients--Family relationships. I. Title.
  RC394.H85S85 2007
  616.8'510092--dc22
  [B]

                                        2006034918

British Library Cataloguing in Publication Data
A CIP catalogue record for this book is available from the British Library

ISBN 978 1 84310 487 2

Printed and Bound in the United States by Thomson-Shore, Inc.

Contents

Thank-yous

Well, I don't want this to sound like Gwyneth Paltrow's Oscar acceptance speech, where she collapsed in tears while thanking the world. But, there are a number of people I just have to mention because they keep us going. First and foremost...

> Thank you to Joanna Davies,
> my incredible friend
> without whom this book would not exist
> and my life would not be nearly as much fun.

Thank you also to:

All at Hightown Surgery who help keep us afloat, particularly Dr Cornwall, Dr Hin and Carol Blake who provide a constant source of insight, wisdom, strength, support and some rather useful medication.

Carol Dutton, our regional advisor for the UK Huntington's Disease Association, who thinks for us, fights for us, argues on our behalf, stands up for us when we are too tired to represent ourselves, finds solutions when we have no ideas or resources of our own left, and generally champions our needs.

My mum, Maggie, who keeps us all going with her constant support, acts as unofficial chauffeur, takes a load off of Phil (everything from keeping Dan in ironed school clothes to Friday afternoon shopping), and keeps coming around to help even when I am snappy and rude to her (sorry about that, Maggie).

Phil's mum, Pat, who lives almost a hundred miles away but regularly makes the journey up to see us, scrubs and irons everything in sight until it gleams and also stays over when Phil has to work away from home.

Caroline, Vicky, John and everyone else at Turpin's Lodge Riding School. And, of course, Charlie, my other man (well, horse, but I tell Phil he's my other man).

My loving friends (you know who you are), especially Helen, Alan and the girls, Andy (Ben) Center, Angela and their girls.

All at the amazing Clive Project (www.thecliveproject.org.uk), who help me live the life I want to live, including Tessa, Nic, Gill and especially, of course, Jo. There are some rare, special people in the world who can light up the lives of those around them. Tess specializes in spotting them and recruits them to work for the Clive Project. It's a unique service and I don't know what I'd do without them.

Introduction: 'The Most Cruel Disease Known to Man'

Huntington disease (HD) is an inherited brain disorder that causes progressive deterioration of the physical, cognitive and emotional self. It leads to severe incapacitation and eventual death 10–40 years after the onset of the disease. Although it usually affects adults between the ages of 30 and 45, symptoms can appear in young children and older adults.

Common symptoms are uncontrollable movements, abnormal balance when walking, slurred speech, difficulty swallowing, thinking difficulties, and personality changes. Each child of an affected parent has a 50% chance of inheriting the HD gene, which is located on chromosome four. There is no cure and no effective treatment exists, but scientists are exploring possible treatments and caregivers are developing new approaches to care.

(Paulsen 1999, p.5)

When people ask us what Huntington's Disease is we say something like 'Imagine the physical effects of Parkinson's Disease, mixed up with the mental deterioration of Alzheimer's and you're in roughly the right territory. It's terminal, but it takes its time, decades sometimes. Oh, and it's hereditary: each of your kids has a 50 per cent chance of inheriting it.'

We've heard Huntington's Disease described as, variously, 'the gradual and relentless dismantling of a human being' (ugh) and 'the most cruel disease known to man' (double ugh).

It's described as 'cruel' because it delivers not just a double whammy, or a triple whammy, but a relentless series of whammies that just keep on hitting a family over the course of years, of generations, in fact.

It just keeps on coming

Steel yourself. There's:

- *a gradual mental decline*, with depression common and pronounced mental illness including psychosis and delusions not uncommon; thought processes decline as the illness gradually kills your brain cells and the connections between them

- *an emotional decline*, leading to sudden mood swings, a blunting of emotions, loss of ability to relate to people you love, frustration, outbursts of anger and aggression

- *physical decline* as you lose control of your muscles, so walking, speaking and eventually swallowing become difficult, things keep dropping to the floor (including you), your arms and legs start moving independently

- *the cumulative effect* being that you usually lose your job, have your driving licence taken away, gradually lose the ability to walk, communicate, eat for yourself, look after other people let alone yourself, think things through properly…all the things you take for granted every day slowly slip away

- *and then there's the ongoing whammy* of worrying whether or not your children and their children will inherit it and start the cycle all over again. The symptoms usually don't appear till early middle-age, so there's an agonizing wait.

Had enough yet? Me too. That's only a select list of symptoms, but I didn't want to hit you with all of them straight away. We're only on the opening pages after all.

Your inclination on reading all that is probably to recoil. It's a bit like being hit by a series of punches from a heavyweight boxer. 'Take this, and that, and this, and that, and…', it just keeps on going. And, when it's done with you, there's the added pain of knowing that it may well start on your kids. It's enough to just make you want to lie flat on the canvas and think, 'What's the point of getting up? It'll just knock me down again'.

But all over the world and throughout history life triumphs because people have refused to stay down when circumstances have knocked them down. You can't stop Huntington's Disease constantly knocking you down – sometimes literally: I've got the bruises to prove it. And it doesn't just knock you down; it knocks whole families down.

Fragmenting families

The illness can seem like a juggernaut ploughing through the family, so massively, awesomely unstoppable that each family member ends up almost paralysed by it; so cowed by its impact or its possible future impact on themselves and on the people they love that they feel powerless to do anything.

The sense of hopelessness HD brings can descend like a cloud on a family. It can freeze love and end up fragmenting that family as everyone runs for cover – either turning in on themselves because the pain of gradually losing yourself and/or the people you love to this relentless illness is too much to bear or, in many cases, physically leaving the family and breaking all contact for the same reasons.

No, you can't stop it knocking you down. After we found out we had Huntington's Disease in our family we got knocked about all over the place by it for a good few years. We were punch drunk, bashed about, reeling. We almost had one or two casualties along the way as one or other of us thought about giving up completely. Careers were derailed, rosy imagined futures disappeared in a puff of smoke. We didn't talk about it unless we absolutely had to. It was the monster in the room everyone tried to ignore, but couldn't.

If you can get through those early years of pain and panic and keep together as a family, you've done well. We are doing better now than in the first few years. And since communication is a great casualty of Huntington's – you can feel that there is nothing positive to say, so you say nothing to each other about it – it's time we talked to each other and to other families who are going through their own tough times, and to people who work with this illness. That is why we have put this book together. Huntington's is a family illness and deserves a family book, one that looks at it from every member of the family's point of view.

An explanatory note: absent voices

The structure of this book is that each member of my core family – my husband, two sons, daughter-in-law and my sister – take a chapter to explain their experience of Huntington's Disease, and to share what we have learnt about how to come to terms with it.

Some people had more time to devote to this than others and so their chapters are longer. That doesn't mean that the shorter chapters are sub-plots with less important stories, just that they were fitted around a full-time college course or job. One or two members of the family – Phil, my husband, in particular – tend to waffle on more than the others. That is reflected in the length of his chapter, too: be warned. His tendency never to use a short sentence when a long one will do might be because when he writes as a journalist he is paid by the word.

There are two people who are central to the story of how we are learning to live with Huntington's Disease in my family, but who do not themselves have a voice in the pages of this book. They are my mother Maggie and my brother Geoff.

Maggie

I did ask Maggie to write a chapter. And she did try, but it was a very upsetting experience for her, raking up years of trauma she had experienced with my dad, Brian, who died of the disease, and then having to explain how she felt on discovering that two of her three children also had the disease. Maggie asked my sister Wendy to write a few words to explain the absence of her chapter. Here's that explanation:

> Throughout the majority of her married life, Mum lived with a violent and abusive man. She had no idea he had Huntington's Disease. They divorced when I was 16, as she could not stand it any more. It was not until years later when we discovered he had HD that she realized why he had been like that. I know from numerous conversations with her that she feels enormous guilt about the fact she did not understand his problems and help him with them, and even greater guilt that two of her children have the gene, though it runs through Dad's not her side of the family.
>
> She is very involved with the local Huntington's Disease group, fund-raising and supporting others who have the illness, and she works tirelessly for any member of the family who needs her.
>
> Everybody who has contributed a chapter to this book has mentioned what a tower of strength Maggie is, and how they would not have coped without her. These chapters were written independently, without collusion, then edited and woven together by Sandy. So it is a testament to Maggie's strength as a person that she appears at the heart of each chapter. She is quite simply amazing, and in effect we have all written her chapter for her. She is so much a part of our lives that none of us could have left her out.

Geoff

My much-loved brother Geoff is 45. A few years ago he took the test for the HD gene and discovered that he has it. His three children are, like my two boys, each 50 per cent at risk of inheriting the illness. For the past couple of years he and I have drifted out of contact, I suspect at least partly because each of us has had to deal with the onset of the symptoms, which can leave you with little energy and inclination to reach out to other people.

I am glad to say that just recently Geoff got back in touch with me again. Unfortunately, it was too late to ask him to contribute his story to this book.

Stronger at the broken places

Huntington's changes everything. But not always for the worse. Danny my younger son, who just turned 15, said the other day, 'I think having Huntington's in the family has made me a better person than I would have been.' I think he's right. It's made us all have to be better people. We've had to rise to it. We've had to find strength we didn't think we had.

Ernest Hemingway wrote, in *A Farewell to Arms*, 'The world breaks everyone and afterward many are strong at the broken places'. We've noticed that each of us has been broken in one way or another by this illness. We are not the same as we were before. It's changed us. Each of us has had to dig deep and go through a private rebuilding of ourselves after finding out Huntington's was in our midst. Not just once, either. It's ongoing. For a while we were fragmented and in disarray. But we have grown back together as a family of individuals who are each stronger than we were before. We are indeed stronger at the broken places.

Sandy Sulaiman

CHAPTER 1

The Eye of the Storm:
Sandy's Story

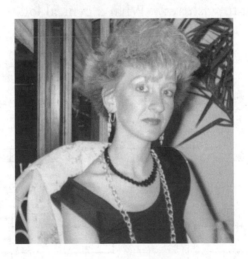

My name is Sandy. I'm 47. I have Huntington's Disease. That sounds like one of those introductions at an Alcoholics Anonymous meeting (I would imagine). I have two boys, Bromley (25) and Danny (15). Each has a 50 per cent chance of inheriting the gene. We'll know one way or the other when they are well into their thirties (probably), as that is usually when the symptoms appear. I myself inherited the Hunting-ton's gene from my dad Brian, who died from the illness in 1995. My brother Geoff also inherited the gene. He's a couple of years younger than me. His three children are therefore also each 50 per cent at risk. Our younger sister Wendy, the baby of the family, did not inherit the gene. Her two girls are, therefore, not at risk of inheriting it as it cannot skip a generation. Phew, some good news to end that introduction with, at least.

Before this chapter starts properly, I need to write you a quick note about my photo. It's me before I developed the symptoms of Huntington's. I wanted you to see me as I am myself, not with any changes that may have been imposed on me by the illness. The rest of the family say this is a ruse to get away with a picture of myself as I was 20 years ago and that in fact it is the change imposed on me by age that I want to wish away. What a cynical lot.

Family tree

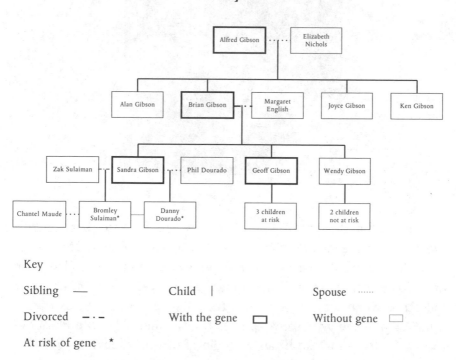

Key

Sibling	—	Child	|	Spouse	......
Divorced	—·—	With the gene	▭	Without gene	▭
At risk of gene	*				

Oh, and a quick explanation of the title of this chapter is needed too, in case it's not obvious. Again according to the rest of the family, I like to sit around relaxing with a cigarette in my hand like some still, small, centre of calm, while they all run around dealing with the fallout of Huntington's Disease. Well, it works for me. So, on we go with my story. I'd like to start with being stuck inside an enormous tube…

Inside the machine

'You'll have to lie still. If you move, it will affect the image and we'll have to do it again,' says a voice. I'm lying on a table. My head is at the opening of a vast, noisy machine. The table, with me on it unfortunately, is about to be sucked into the mouth of the machine. Gulp. I feel like Sean Connery in that James Bond movie where the villain clamps him to a table and the ray from a giant industrial laser is working its way up the table towards him.

'You need to lie still,' repeats the voice gently as my head twitches. 'If I could lie still, I wouldn't need to be here,' I say from my horizontal position. 'Ah, I'd forgotten about your bizarre sense of humour,' smiles the consultant. 'Yes, I do still have one,' I think, while trying not to move. 'Despite the holes in the brain your scanner might show up, wherever my sense of humour is located in there, it's doing a good job of avoiding the damage caused to the rest of my brain by Huntington's.'

That's what Huntington's Disease does to you, gradually destroys brain cells and the connections between them. When you have HD, the medical people like to get a snapshot of your brain as early as possible. They can then compare it with later snapshots (providing you can keep still, I suppose) to see how the disease is progressing.

On this occasion, I was on the table in the MRI Unit (Magnetic Resonance Imager, but you probably knew that already) of Hammersmith Hospital in West London. Dr Puri, the consultant and owner of the disembodied voice, needed a picture of my brain because he was leading a trial for a drug that may help the symptoms of the illness I have. I was one of 100 people taking the trial drug. It was a bit like taking cod liver oil – two light amber-coloured gel capsules taken twice a day. The deal was that if I spent a year on the trial without taking any other medication apart from the anti-depressants, Hormone Replacement Therapy (HRT) tablets and sleeping pills I was on prior to the trial, then I would be rewarded with an endless supply of the drug before it became available to the general public.

The downside was regularly having to go through tests and scans every few months to see how my illness was progressing compared to others on the trial. The trial is over now. The first year was 'blind': half the participants were on placebos and half not. We didn't know which was which. The second year everyone on the trial was on the drug. The trial finished a couple of years ago. We had high hopes at the time for it. But, after two years, the results were not conclusive. There seemed to be a beneficial effect, but it wasn't statistically significant enough to push the drug through the fast track that the Food and Drug Administration in the US and its equivalent in Europe had prepared for it.

So, they are giving it more trials. In the meantime, I keep on taking my free supply. You never know.

Poked and prodded

If you are not careful, life with Huntington's Disease can become a constant round of visits to, or visits by, an endless stream of health and social care professionals. The list has included, at various times: ongoing trips to the family doctor (obviously); a dietician (half a dozen visits); a genetics counsellor (lots of visits); a physiotherapist (one visit was enough); a psychiatrist; an occupational therapist; several consultant doctors specializing in genetics; a movement disorder clinic; various voluntary agencies; social workers; two very nice social care assistants who came to the house wanting to give me a bath – I sent them packing; a neuropsychologist (I think, may have

got that one wrong); a speech therapist whom I didn't actually get
to meet but had several appointments made before she gave up and
sent me a note saying I was no longer on her list…and lots of other
people who tried to intervene in one way or another with varying
degrees of success. Plus the drug trial visits, of course. Oh, and a
homeopathist my sister put me on to, and a faith healer who lives
near my mum, is a very nice lady and helps me feel better by
focusing on colours. There are lots more but that gives you the
general idea.

You have to resist the invasion sometimes. So, quite often, as
with the speech therapist, I just refuse to show up if I'm too worn
out or disinclined to go when the appointment time comes around.
This is known in Huntington's jargon, I believe, as 'challenging
behaviour'. I call it trying to keep some level of control over my life.

Seeing the funny side of things is absolutely essential with Huntington's Disease, as it is with any serious condition. It can surprise
the medical people and is quite useful for getting them to realize
you are a human being, not a lab rat. As anyone who has to make
regular hospital trips to be assessed or for ongoing treatment
knows, medical professionals tend to split into two groups: the ones
who will laugh with you and those who look astonished when you
offer a joke or an opinion, as if they'd assumed you were just a
subject with an interesting condition, not a fully rounded human
with the power of speech.

Sometimes the lack of communication can just be silly. When I
was still able to drive, I had an appointment with a hospital physiotherapist. I had to park quite a way from her building and was a little
late, so ran to get there. She greeted me at the door to her office. I
was panting, having run all the way from reception. 'I don't know
much about Huntington's,' she said immediately. 'Can you walk
unaided?' 'Well, yes, since I'm standing here on my own, and you're
quite a long way from the reception, let alone the car park, and I
gave up flying ages ago, I guess you could say that I can walk

unaided, yes,' I replied. She didn't see the funny side of it. I didn't go back to see her after that. There's that challenging behaviour again. But, you see, my life is shorter than the average. So, I exercise my right to choose whom I spend time with. Would you want to spend one hour a week in a room on your own with a physiothera-pist who has no sense of humour, when the total number of hours you have at your disposal for the rest of your life is pretty precious to you?

Anyway, I've always been challenging, with or without Hun-tington's Disease. Let's look back a bit to prove it.

Before Huntington's

If we roll back time, even further than that ancient picture of me at the start of this chapter, we come to my early childhood in Whitley Bay, Northumberland, north-east England. It was a lovely time (aren't most early childhood memories?) enjoying the usual child-hood pursuits, visiting the beach, having picnics at the seaside and playing with my friends. I was the oldest of three and apparently the most obnoxious and outspoken even then. I remember being sent to my room once by my mum and spending the afternoon sitting on my bed and quietly peeling the wallpaper off the wall behind it.

When I was 12 we moved south, following my dad's work, to live in a small village called Ledwell in Oxfordshire. Actually, it is so small it's not technically a village but a hamlet, just a collection of houses. I went to the local comprehensive at the nearby town of Chipping Norton, where I quickly learnt to lose my Geordie accent from the north-east, on pain of death or, worse, public humiliation through teasing. I was good at English, like my journalist dad, and also loved art and drama. I was small but noisy – challenging even then, you see – and it was hard to get me to shut up in school. An inspired drama teacher decided to channel the loud voice and inces-sant talking by getting me to play Eliza Doolittle in the school play *Pygmalion*. I thought about pursuing a career in acting but didn't fancy being unemployed for great lengths of time and never was very good at waiting on tables.

The most significant part of my life at that time was that I had a pony, a Welsh mountain breed called Jingle. As I have become less mobile in recent years, and am no longer able to drive, I have gone back to those happy teen years in one way, by taking up riding again. Renewing my love affair with horses (specifically, Charlie, whom I ride at least twice a week) is great exercise and does the job of visiting a physiotherapist, in my opinion, with one improvement: Charlie has a better sense of humour.

Just to prove I had a life before Huntington's Disease, forgive me while I gallop (ahem) through the next few stages of that life before HD. I wanted to be a journalist like my dad. So, I left home and headed for the big city, where I attended the London College of Fashion to study fashion journalism. My dad had often taken me to London to meet BBC colleagues and to take me out filming and so the big city was familiar to me. I lived in Queensway, near Hyde Park. I walked to college each day because I was so broke. I lived in the Methodist International Hostel, which was for students who had a connection with the Methodist Church. There were lots of students from around the world. I loved living there.

Following in Dad's footsteps

My diploma course in fashion journalism lasted one year and then I became a journalist. So far, all was going according to plan. At the John Lewis Partnership, my second employer, I was assistant editor on three papers. I think I was one of the youngest ever section managers there, at 19.

By the time I was 21, the plan was off. I had acquired over the previous two years, not necessarily in this order, one son, Bromley and one husband, Zak. The former I kept. The latter didn't work out quite so well. I went back to university to study for a degree in sociology. Brom went to a childminder, who would later on become my mother-in-law, though of course I did not know it at the time!

While I was studying for my degree I fell in love with Phil, who had just left university, was teaching English as a foreign language, and was living upstairs in his parents' house. I met Phil in the early 1980s. They were carefree times. We ended up in a band together called the Bronsons. Phil played the drums and I sang backing vocals (badly). We played in pubs and clubs at night while working as press officers during the day.

When we both hit 30, I heard from my dad, who hadn't been a part of my life for many years (it will become clear why as you read the rest of this book). He wrote to tell me he had been diagnosed with a possibly hereditary illness. It was an incorrect diagnosis, as it turned out, of an illness that would leave him in a wheelchair, and that would eventually do the same to me if I inherited it. It was shocking information and made us reassess our lives.

We both decided to be more adventurous instead of slipping into middle-age with deskbound jobs as press officers. We gave up our jobs, and headed off to California for several months. The plan was that we would both become freelance journalists. There is a strong demand among UK newspapers and magazines for 'only in America'-type stories. What happens in America first the UK catches up with later. So, to spot stories to sell to English magazines and newspapers it made sense to spend some time over there, with access to stories the UK-based freelances we were competing against didn't have. It meant very little income and very big outgoings for a few months. It was a gamble. But 'no pain, no gain' as Jane Fonda used to say in that decade.

It also meant no school for a couple of months for Bromley, as we taught him on the road. He seemed quite happy with that. When we came back we started to work as freelance journalists writing for national newspapers and magazines. Phil and I were married in 1991 after ten years of living together. I was pregnant with my second son Danny. We lived in Chiswick, West London for about five years and then, after Danny was born, we moved to Oxfordshire. Our freelance careers had both taken off successfully. I wrote for most of the national newspapers as well as magazines such as *Mother & Baby, Fashion Weekly, Options* and *Bella*. I wrote articles largely about childcare and women's issues. Both Phil and I worked mainly from home so that we could look after the kids.

We even worked on some articles together. One interesting article I wrote was about men's attitudes to women who drive flash cars. We persuaded Mazda to let me have an MX5 roadster (they call it the Miata in the US) for a week. I drove around in it while Phil sat low down in the passenger seat with a notebook taking notes about how men drivers reacted to a blonde at the wheel of a sporty-looking car. It did indeed seem true that, as we had suspected, men became more competitive and aggressive drivers if they encountered a woman in a sports car.

I even did live radio interviews based on my articles. Phil said I was fearless as he hates live interviews and would only do them if recorded. It didn't bother me. On one occasion a radio station asked me to talk on air about the Mazda sports car experiment and put me up against the aggressive (very male) motoring journalist Jeremy Clarkson. After he had said, 'The car you chose for your experiment isn't a real sports car anyway. It's a hairdresser's car,' I think I won. I inadvertently called him Jeremy Paxman instead of Clarkson and he became slightly flustered as the presenter couldn't stop laughing.

That was then, this is now

Phil, my husband, says I tend to gloss over some of the difficult things about these years I've just described. You'll need to read his chapter for a slightly alternative view of how our life was progressing at this time. The main revelation to hit us during those years was when we found out my dad had Huntington's Disease, not the cerebellar ataxia he had been diagnosed with.

When we were told, it meant very little. My husband found the number for and called the Huntington's Disease Association, desperate to find out what the implications were. The first hint we had then about how hard it can be to deal with the information about this illness was that, oddly it seemed to us at the time, they wouldn't give us any over the phone! Phil was almost shouting at them down the phone saying, 'Just give me some basic information now, please. You can imagine how anxious we are to know exactly what this is.' There was no broadband giving fast internet access then, so that wasn't an option.

The person at the end of the phone said the information could be so devastating that she couldn't give it out, that we needed to talk to someone who had been trained and could give us the information in the least damaging way. It seemed bizarre at the time. In fact, on reflection, it still seems bizarre, but I guess they need to make absolutely sure you don't give someone the wrong information. They put some leaflets in the post and we were hit with it a couple of days later: the fact that it is hereditary, that there is a 50 per cent inheritance risk, that there is no cure, it is terminal, affects you physically and mentally, involves a relentless slow decline in all your faculties, and that, as the icing on the cake, doctors refer to it as 'the cruellest disease known to man'.

For a few months we were reeling, as this illness has so many elements to it that we had to absorb and come to terms with – your parent being terminally ill, yourself being at risk, your children being at risk, too; what to tell and not to tell the children: it was as if our lives were unravelling. Then my dad went on to die of the disease. We saw at first hand how it can dismantle someone.

Anyway, life was about to change completely.

Finding out I have the disease

A couple of years after my dad died I was on a course at Oxford Brookes University, training to become a lecturer in journalism.

That's when I first had to face the fact that I had indeed inherited Huntington's Disease. By then we knew that this was the illness my dad had had. We had spent a lot of time, described elsewhere in this book, helping him get into a care home before he died. I knew I was 50 per cent at risk of inheriting the illness. I had chosen not to take the genetic test which would tell me if I had the gene or not.

I was giving a presentation of a lesson plan, when my tutor pulled me aside and pointed out to me that I shouldn't wear brace-lets, because my movements made them jangle and create too much noise. She said I appeared to have 'a motor problem' and asked me what it was. I was devastated, as I had not noticed any symptoms myself. I burst into tears and explained, between sobs, that my father had died of Huntington's Disease and the movements she described were a symptom, so I must have inherited it, too.

It was then I decided teaching would be too stressful a job for me and I gave up the course. When I came home from the college session where the lecturer had pointed out my movements to me, I was obviously devastated. I was in tears – I don't know how I drove the 20 miles from Oxford to Bloxham, the village where we live, in that state. My husband Phil sat me down, made me a cup of tea, and asked me to tell him what was wrong. When I told him what had happened, his face fell.

I went on to discover later that Phil knew that I had the illness but hadn't felt able to tell me. I had made it clear at the time that I didn't want the blood test, as there is no cure. The majority of people don't want to know. If there was a cure obviously that would be different.

The blood test – confirming it for sure

The worst fear is the fear of the diagnosis – not knowing. So, the five years or so knowing I had a 50 per cent chance of inheriting it had been full of worry. A needle pricking my finger was the first step in finding out for sure that I had Huntington's Disease. The neurologist then undertook several co-ordination tests on me, similar to when the police test motorists to see if they are drunk. You'll be familiar with this from the movies. Or, perhaps from your own experience. You have to touch your nose, walk in a straight line and so on.

For some reason, having been quite stoical up to this point, I suddenly found this process horrible. I felt humiliated. Phil was there with me and confirmed afterwards what I thought as I went through what I came to think of as an ordeal. The doctor was blunt, cold and clinical. I felt I was being treated more as a lab assessment, a curiosity or a clinical exercise than a person.

I had to wait an agonizing month for the blood test results and when they arrived I had to go back to the hospital to see the same cold and clinical neurologist as before. She said, 'Bad news…', and went on to tell me I not only had the Huntington's gene, but that my reactions to the cognitive and movement tests showed I had the symptoms as well. When I found out, it was actually a relief to know, in a bizarre kind of way. My view had been, over the seven previous years during which we had learnt about HD and seen its effects on my dad, that if I knew I had it, I wouldn't be able to live with that knowledge. That's what I told my husband whenever we discussed having the test. But, as often happens when you have shocking news, you don't react the way you think you would. You find strength from somewhere. After a cursory 'We would advise people in your situation not to have any more children,' which I interpreted as 'We don't want any more like you around, do we,' we went home.

Telling the children

Lots of couples who know they have Huntington's in their families choose not to have children in case they inherit it. I already had two sons when I found out. But I don't regret having them. I'm glad for many reasons that I did not have to make that choice. I like to think my choice would have been the same. I have no regrets at all. Both my sons are the best things that happened to me. I love being a mum. I couldn't imagine a world without them.

I was 41 when diagnosed with the illness. Both my sons, Bromley (now 25) and Danny (now 15), have had to learn to live with the fact that not only will they lose their mother to this illness – unless the high living I engage in gets me first. I'm doing my best. That's a joke, by the way. But they also have had to adapt to the fact that there is a 50 per cent chance that either or both of them might have inherited the defective gene from me.

I had already told them we had Huntington's in our family. You'd be surprised how many people in our situation don't. Some families don't talk about it because it's too painful, or they feel defeated by it. A parent's natural instinct is to protect their children, perhaps by withholding information. But we should never underestimate our children's capacity to cope, particularly with information like this.

Research shows that it is, in fact, better to be honest about it as early as possible, because children find it harder to deal with the shock of discovering they or their family are 'different' later in childhood than if they have known about it for as long as they can remember.

Developing the symptoms

When I first started to develop the symptoms of Huntington's, I didn't try to hide them, though it is easy to feel self-conscious as it affects one's movement, concentration and memory. When I am tired I forget words in the middle of sentences, which is particularly frustrating for me as a writer and because I have always had a very good memory. I realized that I was forgetting little details that normally I remembered, such as...er, I forget where that sentence was going. Yes, that was for dramatic effect. Sorry about that. I also get angry and frustrated about things that normally wouldn't have affected me.

The symptoms take hold progressively over a 10- to 15-year period, so it's a gradual decline. People with Huntington's are often accused of being drunk, because of the combination of slurred speech and a tendency to fall over! The illness affects my balance and co-ordination. Though I find it difficult I can still walk at the moment. People in the latter stages of the illness can't, so often they have to use a wheelchair.

I can't protect them from it

I know that if either of the boys do get it, there will be nothing I can do to protect them or help them, as I probably won't be around. Any mother's natural instinct is to protect their children and it is hard to imagine that situation, and also that the illness would have come down through me. So I try to live a full and active life, and to be as positive and cheerful as possible. If I can make it clear I value and enjoy every minute of time I am with them, it shows them that if they do get it, life goes on. That's the best thing I can do for them.

Involuntary movements are just one of the symptoms of my illness. Losing weight, due to the energy taken up by the continuous involuntary movements, is a problem for people with Huntington's. So, I am on a high-calorie diet (the envy of most women I know). I can eat whatever I like, and do! From fry-ups to Chinese food to ice-cream, my eating habits are the envy of my friends. As Hunting-ton's is a disease of the brain I make a point of eating food such as fish, cod liver oil and blueberries, all reputedly good 'brain food'.

It is dreadful to be always dropping and breaking things. I can't cook any more, which is why Phil does it. We always shared mundane tasks like housework, ironing and cooking, but now he has to do all of that, with the help of an occasional cleaner plus my mum and his own mum coming in to help to stop things getting on top of him, as I find these things too difficult.

I can only concentrate on one thing at a time; this is a symptom of Huntington's and multi-tasking has become impossible. Also my tiredness is a problem; I've always had lots of energy but by the early afternoon these days, I can feel exhausted. I am much slower in my ability to think and make decisions – I used to write fast and think fast, but I can't do this now. I was very decisive.

I will be on anti-depressants and sleeping pills for the rest of my life. When I don't take the anti-depressants I lose interest in life, everything seems pointless, I feel lethargic and obviously if I'm depressed it affects my concentration. I've always had a very good sense of direction, but as the Huntington's developed I found that I was getting lost more when I was driving.

Sleeping through the earthquake

I also used to be a really heavy sleeper. When we were working in California I slept through an earthquake in San Francisco that had woken Phil up and made all the newspaper front pages the next day. I even slept through the famous 1987 hurricane in England. But sleeping now can be difficult, which is why I am on sleeping pills. I can't remember my dreams any more, oddly, and I used to have nice ones!

It could be easy to be self-conscious as I do drop things in shops. People tend not to intrude too much which is good. I can't read my own handwriting any more. I originally said 'No thanks' to a disabled badge for my car because I felt like a fraud. But, more recently, after losing the right to drive and having to be driven around everywhere, I have had to accept a disabled parking disc for whoever is driving me around at the time.

Losing my independence

When you are forced to face something inevitable like this, there's an initial period of shock and disbelief, anger, fear, a sense that your life is over. But you either collapse and take to your bed, or you keep getting back up every time the illness progresses a bit more and knocks you back. Like when I was told I could no longer drive.

I lost my licence after suffering from Huntington's for a couple of years. You don't legally have to tell your employers if you have a disease but you do legally have to tell the driving licence authority in the UK and the car insurance company. I had to take an annual driving assessment, which seemed to me harder than the original driving test itself. It's a serious point, actually. If 'ordinary' people had to retake their driving test every year, how many of them would pass every time?

I twice took the assessment. I passed the test the first year. But, the second time, a year later, even though everyone thought I would pass, I failed. When the man conducting the test told me I'd failed, it was a major change to my life and I felt everything crashing down around my ears. I couldn't nip to the shops any time I wanted, visit friends, go clothes shopping, pick the boys up from school if they needed it…all the things you take for granted. In a stroke of his pen in the 'failed' box, the world in which I could operate independently had suddenly shrunk to the house and how far I could walk from there. And walking wasn't getting any easier.

So I stormed out, leaving him standing there in the reception area of the test centre. He was trying to say some consoling words, but anything he said after the words 'I'm sorry, you've failed' were a blur. I just had to get out of there. I was so shocked and furious at having my independence taken away. I just hadn't expected it at all. I remember staggering outside, fumbling for a cigarette, with tears of anger in my eyes. I instantly lost my freedom to drive and Phil had to bring me home. You can't appeal. That's it. No more car.

This loss of freedom and independence was really hard for me to deal with. From that moment on I had to rely on everybody else for lifts. After being able to drive myself to Oxford to buy clothes, to London to see friends, even do mundane tasks like visiting a super-

'market, I found myself stuck in the middle of the countryside in Oxfordshire, with no means of transport but the local bus service. I had spotted one bus in the ten years or so we had lived there.

My work suffered too. After I was diagnosed with Huntington's, I continued to write a few articles but I found the ability to carry on writing, to the degree I had done before diagnosis, increasingly hard to maintain. I think the shock of finding out I had Huntington's dampened much of my creative capability and I also suffered from extreme tiredness, which affected my capacity to write. Having said that, I did write a few articles for different papers about my battle with this disease. Realistically though, Huntington's pretty much ended my writing career.

There have been so many misunderstandings about Huntington's. Most people in the UK had never heard of it until recently, when it was featured on the TV soap opera EastEnders, where it was presented in such a negative way, with the introduction of a character in the final stages of the illness, bed-bound, helpless and unable to speak. That's not me.

My rather cynical theory about why HD has such a low profile is that no one famous has died of Huntington's, apart from Woody Guthrie, the American folk singer. In our celebrity-obsessed society, people like Michael J. Fox and Ronald Reagan have raised awareness of Parkinson's and Alzheimer's, respectively. But we in the HD community lack a celebrity sufferer. There is ongoing genetic research into this disease but unfortunately there is no cure at the moment. I think the drug trial I took part in possibly helped with some of the symptoms.

Live life to the full: the positives

Nowadays, after years of adjusting, I try not to think about my illness but rather to concentrate on what I can do. I spend much of my time at a local riding school, having taken up horse riding again after many years. It was a passion of mine – I had a pony as a teenager, as I mentioned above. And I found it's a hobby I still can˙ do. My body just seems to remember how to control the horse, Caroline, the owner of the stables where I ride, told me. She had been concerned my movements – my arms and body muscles tend to move constantly – would confuse the horse. But they turned out not to and so I have rediscovered a skill and passion I had not found the time to keep involved with. And I am grateful to her for giving me the chance to try and prove I could do it.

A couple of years ago I got it into my head that there was one thing I needed to replace my little sporty car that had been taken away. It was taken away shortly after I opened the driver's door into the path of a car coming up behind me and as the car passed it virtually ripped the door off. The car couldn't be economically repaired and shortly after that I failed my test. What I needed to win back some independence, I realized, was my own horse.

Phil almost had a heart attack (that would have helped pay for a horse, actually – he's nicely insured, whereas my life can't be because of the Huntington's). He came up with all kinds of arguments as to why we couldn't afford to buy and then maintain a horse. He used words like 'maintain' as if it was a car. My sister Wendy came to the rescue with a creative solution just as I was about to find something really heavy with which to convince Phil that, compared to a number of blows around the head, the cost of a horse was painless. That's a joke too, by the way. Wendy's solution was a rent-a-horse scheme where you can ride a horse a certain number of times a week for a monthly fee. We found our local stables, Turpin's Lodge, offered this 'horse for hire' type of programme and tried it for six months.

It was brilliant, but I wanted more. I still wanted my own horse. Phil and I clashed a few times more over this. Then Caroline at the stable came up with yet another creative solution. One of her horses, Charlie, who happened to be my regular ride and whom I loved dearly, was due to retire. They would keep him on for a year or two and treat him as mine for that time if we paid the livery (that's his upkeep, vet's bills, food and so on). This is hugely therapeutic for me and I try to ride at least once a week. I have fallen off a lot, but I always get back on eventually!

Another plus thing to come out of not being able to drive, as well as rediscovering riding, is I have a great new friend called Jo from an organization called the Clive Project, who pops around twice a week. Jo says her job is partly to make my dreams come true; to find out what I want to do in life and act as my facilitator to make it happen. She is amazingly good at it! I enjoy the freedom and independence this gives me and the sense of being in control. The fresh air and exercise of riding helps me counter depression and is good for balance and co-ordination. On a broader level, Jo simply makes my life richer and I look forward to her coming over.

The family counts

We make a point of taking more family holidays together – conscious of the fact that time together as a family is more precious as it is likely to be shorter than for most people. I love the adventure of visiting new places and different cultures. One unexpected positive thing about my diagnosis is that we now, as a family, take adventurous holidays that we might otherwise have postponed until later life, including a trip to Southern Australia a couple of years ago, where we met the in-laws – my son Bromley married a lovely Australian girl, Chantel – and travelled the Great Ocean Road in a rickety old motor-home.

Phil now works from home so he can be around to keep me company and we can do things together, like nipping out to the local pubs for lunch. I get far more tired than I used to, so he has gradually taken over some things that we used to split 50–50, like making sure our younger son has clean clothes for school and someone to see him off in the morning, shopping and stuff – my mum pops around to help with things, too. He helps me deal with all the social services, health professionals and other bureaucracy that crops up when you have a disabling illness. And he picks me up when I fall over.

Not fade away

I realize that through my diagnosis of Huntington's I have lost my future. I will not live to be old. I suppose that I have always known, certainly since my dad was diagnosed with Huntington's, that the outlook for me was quite bleak. I live with this by distracting myself, I suppose. Phil helped me cash in my small employee's pension recently because I felt that I should be able to enjoy the benefits of it now rather than when it is too late, because I'm not going to make retirement. Phil now tells me it has all gone on paying for Charlie for two years and on covering the cost of my cigarettes. I'm not sure I believe him. He's swanning around in a rather expensive-looking shirt at the moment. I'll have to hunt out the receipt and see if I'm paying for it. That's another joke, by the way.

My dad didn't make it to his 60th. He died when he was 59. When you know you won't live to be old, memories are more important than material things. I love doing things together as a family, spending time with the people I love, celebrating Christmas and birthdays and heading off on family holidays. We drag all the family away with us at least once a year, whether they like it or not.

Though I have this disease I will not let it overwhelm me. I intend to live my life to the full, to enjoy every day, spend happy times with my children and the people I love, plus Charlie the horse. I am not going to go quietly into that still night, or whatever the phrase is. I am going to continue being as noisy and challenging as possible. I still bleach my hair. Yas, my brilliant hairdresser, still spikes it up and makes it look pretty formidable for me. Challenging behaviour has always been my speciality. I see no reason to stop now.

CHAPTER 2

The Lucky One?
The Sister's Story

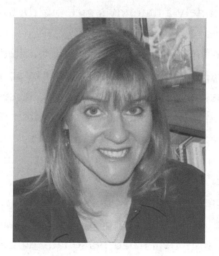

I am Sandy's sister Wendy. Sandy is seven years older than me. So, from her point of view, as she was growing up, I was her annoying little sister. Geoff, our brother, is between us age-wise, which helped reduce the clashes we had. When Sandy left home at 18, she and I became friends (we weren't when we were younger) and ended up having babies within seven weeks of each other: her second and my first child. That was a great time in my life; we were so close. I was tested for HD in 1997 and I do not have the gene. So, I am the lucky one of the three of us. I will not get the illness, and neither will my kids. My husband and mum will not have to watch me become more and more ill and unable to do all the things I love to do. I am the lucky one, aren't I?

About Dad

I grew up in a strange household. On one hand we were very lucky. Dad had a good job, we lived in a big house and had (on the surface) all the material things you could want. But the flip side was Dad. He was so unpredictable, one minute loving and fun, the next yelling and abusive. Sandy once told me I never really knew Dad, because by the time I arrived, he had changed. She was always much closer to him. I was definitely a mummy's girl, but then she was safe and consistent. He wasn't.

My teens were the worst. Thankfully he worked in Kuwait so we did not have to see much of him. When Mum and Dad eventually split up, I felt massive relief; I wouldn't have to see him any more. Then he wrote and told me that if I wanted him to continue paying parental maintenance, I had to meet him every time he was in the UK and write to him while he was in Kuwait. I had no choice. We could not live without his money.

I did as he asked, and it was pure hell. When we met, he would spend all the time we were together telling me that the awful things he used to do, things that I had personally witnessed, had never happened. Mum had made it all up to make him look bad. I was 17, and my brain was being tied into knots. If it hadn't been for Mum, I would be a total wreck. She kept me sane; she told me we didn't need the money that badly and that nothing was worth being treated like this. As soon as I turned 18 I cut him off completely and had nothing to do with him for many years.

Learning you are at risk

My older daughter was a year old when we found out Dad had Huntington's Disease. Sandy knew first, but delayed telling me so I could enjoy my daughter's first birthday. A week or so later she broke the news to me. It didn't seem too major a deal at the time. He had previously been diagnosed with cerebellar ataxia, so a new diagnosis of yet another illness we had heard very little about was not too daunting. But, after a visit to my doctor to find out more, things slowly began to sink in.

I realized that I might not be around to watch my daughter grow up. I might not be at her wedding. I remember taking her to a fair and acting as if everything I did with her would be the last time. I wanted her to have such a great day that she would always remember me like this, her mum, full of life and happy.

Although I remember certain things about those years when I was at risk of inheriting Huntington's, my defence mechanism is to forget. Just as I had managed to forget all the awful things that happened in my childhood. You don't really forget, of course. You just blank them out, as it is too painful to live with constantly recurring memories of the violence, the drinking and the fights. The one question that always stuck with me as I was growing up was 'Why is my dad not like other people's?' I just thought he was an awful person. Even with the diagnosis of HD I could not suddenly wipe those years away and say, 'It wasn't him, it was the disease'. I am afraid it does not work like that for me.

So, I didn't really have a dad. Lots of people don't. But to me it didn't really matter that much, because I had a loving mum, a brother and, as I grew older, a relationship with my sister. I know Sandy would agree that we did not get on in the early years. She was seven years older than me and I was the annoying baby sister. It was only after she left home at 18 that we became friends.

My brother Geoff

My brother Geoff was (is) everything to me. He took me everywhere with him, and protected me from the worst of our parents' fights. As he grew older, he was able to step in physically and protect my mum from my dad, which he sometimes had to do. He was good looking, popular, kind, gentle and loving. He was everything to me and the only decent male role model in my life. Nothing could defeat him…except HD.

Another of my rare Huntington's memories is the day Geoff told me he had the gene. I knew he was getting tested, but I was so sure my amazing brother could not be ill that I did not fear the result. When he told me on the phone that the test was positive, I remember being very strong for him and saying all the right things. But, as soon as I put the phone down I literally crumpled to the floor. I howled and screamed. The truest, strongest person in my life had been taken away from me. There was no justice in that. Now my brother was going to be lost to this horrible disease. I knew, even though he had no symptoms as yet, he would never be the same person again. A blow like that changes your whole outlook on life, and he would have to change to adapt to the information he had now been given regarding his future. Geoff had always been there for me; I would now be there for him when he needed support and comfort. Although he lives some distance from me, I have always been ready to go to him, he only has to ask.

Meeting Dad again

You cannot live a normal life with so much grief and anger constantly on the surface. So I shut it down. Very few people ever saw how it affected me. I don't think that is a very healthy way of living, but at the time it was my only way of coping. Dad and I were brought back together after he tried to commit suicide. He had been living in London for a few years (Sandy kept me up to date with his whereabouts). She rang me to say he had been taken into hospital and might not make it.

I went with her to visit. He looked so old and broken, just a frail impersonation of the big bullying person I remembered. He could no longer hurt me. He survived the overdose and was committed to a psychiatric ward. I did what I do best, looked at all the practical issues, and helped to sort them out.

Sandy, Geoff and I spent a whole day clearing his flat, which was full of evidence of his paranoia, spanning right back to our childhood days. He had obviously been ill even then. They say HD symptoms do not come on until later in life (usually) but I think if you know where to look there is evidence of the illness even when the person is called asymptomatic or supposedly not showing any symptoms. In Sandy's case, the family joke was always that she could not walk in a straight line: Mum would say she had a list to starboard. In Dad's case it was the paranoia.

Among the boxes of papers we cleaned out of his flat were copies of old letters that gave us some insight into Dad's thinking over the years. There were exchanges of letters making it clear he had been sacked from a number of jobs. This is a common pattern with Huntington's as people become inflexible, stubborn, often aggressive and unable to co-operate with their co-workers. But Dad had kept all these sackings a secret. He used to storm home shouting to Mum about how he had quit because so-and-so was unbearable to work with. We didn't realize how many jobs he had lost till we found those letters.

There was also a whole file of angry (on his side) correspondence with his old employers, the BBC, including many complaining of a vendetta against Dad to prevent him becoming Director-General – the top job at the BBC that he had felt was naturally his, according to the letters, but that had been kept from him. Dad worked at the BBC for many years and achieved pretty senior positions, but was never in line for that level of job.

One copy of a letter we found gave us quite a shock. It was a character reference for a friend of Dad's who was applying for a job. The letter read like a perfectly normal reference, full of praise for his friend's diligence, capacity for hard work, good track record when she had worked for him and all the usual stuff. Then the last sentence, written in perfect deadpan style so you had to read it twice before it sank in, simply said, 'In fact, if she could conquer her drink problem, which she will never do, she would be the perfect employee.'

If the original was ever sent it was a terrible piece of sabotage to someone's career. Reading it out of context it was shocking but incredibly funny at the same time. But mixed in with the shock that made us laugh at the letter as we handed it to each other in disbelief was an underlying sadness at the reminder of the casual cruelty that this illness can bring out in people, and the damage that casual cruelty causes to others.

Duty not love

As Dad became more ill with the HD, I channelled my energies into helping him. He was in a nursing home by now, so I would visit him as often as I could. I am ashamed to say it was out of duty, not love. Too much had happened in the past for me to be able to say I loved him.

My husband David and I decided to have another child, not an easy decision when you know you might get this awful disease, and worse still pass it on to someone else. I had not had the genetic test to see if I had the Huntington's gene at that stage.

Then Dad died suddenly of pneumonia. I felt nothing. All my emotions towards him had been anaesthetized over the years. I was visiting a friend in the US when I was told the news. I remember spending the rest of the week with my friend, thinking, 'My dad has just died, I should be devastated.' Life was too painful, so it was best to stop feeling anything at all. Of course, this is not humanly possible, so instead of feeling emotion about the big things in life, I would get very angry over tiny little things. I would kick the wall and knock big chunks out of it when my baby would not sleep, or throw the bin across the kitchen when I realized I had left a bag of shopping in town.

This led to me then panicking that I was becoming violent, so therefore I must have HD, and I would spiral down and down. My emotions swung like a pendulum. There was never a happy medium. Anyone at risk from HD will recognize these thought processes; the fear that lives with you daily.

Being unable to grieve

I felt guilty for not loving my dad, and not being able to grieve for him. I am normally such a sensitive person; this lack of emotion was really out of character. I went back to my genetics counsellor, Ruth. She helped me through it as best she could, but nothing could change the past. Over the years, I have slowly learnt to live with my lack of feelings, and although this may sound really weird I have formed a bond with him now he is dead. I know now that he did not mean to mess me up as much as he did, and I believe he is often with me, especially when I am writing, as I have started to do a bit lately, for my work (Dad was a journalist and writing was his passion). Real or not, this comforts me.

As a family, we decided to take Dad's ashes back to Whitley Bay, by the sea on England's north-east coast where we grew up, and scatter them around St Mary's lighthouse, which stands on an outcrop and can be reached from the beach. It was the best and worst weekend. The best because here I was with my mum, sister and brother (plus his small daughter); four of the people I love best in the world. Geoff and I shared the driving. We had such a great time, visiting our old house, schools and stomping grounds, sharing stories about our life. It was therapeutic and bonding.

But it was the worst because every time I was the passenger in the back, sitting next to Sandy, I realized that she was constantly fidgeting. She seemed unable to keep still. People with Huntington's constantly move. My suspicions grew over the weekend. When we got back from the trip, and I was dropping Mum off at her house, I cornered her and gently told her my suspicions. She said she had experienced the same thing when sitting next to Sand. We both knew the worst; Sandy had HD.

Suddenly, the disease had taken my sister away from me too.

Truth is the first casualty

Her husband, Phil, confirmed it. He had known for a while, but we were advised not to tell her as she did not seem ready to face it, particularly while she was still grieving for her dad. Until she had got past the trauma of Dad's death, which seemed to be hitting her very hard, it would be unhelpful for her to have the fact that she herself had HD thrown in her face.

And so began the years of not-telling-Sandy. Everything became secretive, whispered, coming up with and then changing stories so she would not know how people were helping her in the background. I believe this is a part of the illness; HD breeds secrecy and distorts the truth. I could not bear to think that this could happen to me. I would have hated people constantly guessing has she/hasn't she? So I went back to Ruth and asked for the test.

God's dice

The test is preceded by more genetic counselling to prepare you. But, again, I'm afraid my memory fails me. My protective mechanism has kicked in and I can remember very little of this time. David and I both went for the counselling. I was asked how I would feel if I did not have the gene, knowing as I did that Geoff and Sandy did have it.

Apparently, many people in my situation feel huge guilt. But I did not see it that way. I obviously had no control over how I was conceived and whether the HD gene came with that conception or was left out. Similarly, I did not sell out my brother and sister by ensuring they got the gene so I might not get it. None of it was my fault. None of it is anyone's fault. It is pure chance.

I cannot remember very much else of the counselling, but I had to wait seven months before I was allowed the test itself. When that sunny July day dawned, I was more nervous than I had ever been in my life. David drove me to the Churchill Hospital, Oxford. We had been advised to tell as few people as possible that I was having the test so that, if I changed my mind at the last minute, no one would ask awkward questions. No one except David knew what I was doing, which was very strange as I always shared so much with Mum. But this time she was the last person I wanted to know, as I did not want her to worry, and she was also the person I dreaded giving the result to, in case I had to tell her all of her children had the gene.

I remember David parking the car, and me being unable to keep still; walking round and round in a tight circle while he got a ticket from the machine. I remember the doctor and Ruth being there, and I remember the doctor going to get the results from the lab. They do not look at the results in advance. They wait until you confirm that you really want to know. Then they go and get them. This way they cannot accidentally break the news to you if you change your mind.

I remember him coming back into the room to tell me I did not have the gene. In that moment, that doctor was the most perfect person in the world. I felt pure love for him. He had given me and my children such a huge gift. But of course he hadn't really, because he had not given me back my dad, my childhood, my brother, my sister and my future with them.

I should be so lucky

When the topic of this hereditary illness comes up in conversations, and you tell people about the 50 per cent inheritance rate and that you can be tested to see if you will inherit it, people always want to know your status. Some ask outright, others hedge. I usually tell them up front, 'I don't have the gene'. The reaction is always 'So, you turned out to be the lucky one, then.' I sometimes agree with them. It is easier than having to explain that no one who has HD in their family is 'lucky'. No one escapes the illness. No one is exempt. There is no free pass allowing you out of the Huntington's club. We all have to deal with it in one way or another.

Dealing with losing three members of your family is not easy. On bad days, when I am feeling really uncharitable, I even feel like I have lost my mum, as she is so concerned about Sandy and Geoff and what is going on for them that I want to say, 'What about me? Can we have one day when we don't have to think about how HD has ripped our family apart?'

That is totally unfair, but then so is HD. Before the diagnoses we were a close unit, Mum, Sand, Geoff and me. We had survived living with an aggressive husband/father, and that drew us together. We thought that was the end, we could move on and heal. Unfortunately, it was just the beginning.

This may sound as though I live my life feeling sorry for myself, but of course I don't. These thoughts are not constant ones, just the ones that get me when I am feeling down. The majority of the time I am fine and enjoy life. But neither can I pretend that everything is hunkydory and I have accepted the illness and its implications. There is always a polarity to everything in the universe; we all live with conflicting and contradictory emotions.

The person or the disease?

I often look at things in terms of the disease or the person, trying to find the dividing line between the two. For example, Sandy and I had a big falling out a few years ago. I explained it to myself by thinking, 'Well, she wouldn't have been like that if she didn't have Huntington's. It is the disease that makes her like that.'

Actually, it is not as simple as that. Even before I knew of HD it was there in the family, shaping us and our future, working silently in the background (or in Dad's case not so silently). When the Huntington's gene is in your family, there is no 'life before Huntington's' and 'life after Huntington's', which is the way we all neatly try to separate our lives out to make sense of it. Huntington's weaves its way into people's lives bit by bit, affecting individuals who have the gene long before the symptoms actually come out, and affecting the relationships between us in subtle ways as well as in the big, full-blown aggressive ways that come with a diagnosis and the 'official' symptoms.

I think I will have really accepted Huntington's disease and its effect on my family when I can honestly say that my sister and brother are who they are, rather than explaining certain behaviour as being 'down to the HD, not them' and other behaviour being 'more like them'.

Maybe it is because I am removed (and sometimes I do deliberately remove myself) from the day to day reality of HD, that I am not able to accept it as much as other family members. Or maybe I am still that annoying little sister, the youngest child who can't always get her own way. But having a tantrum and running to Mum will not help me this time. My family has HD and I have to live with it the best way I know how. Most of the time I do manage that and get on with life. But, the lucky one? I don't think so. Never once have I considered myself to be the lucky one.

CHAPTER 3

Lost and Found:
The Older Son's Story

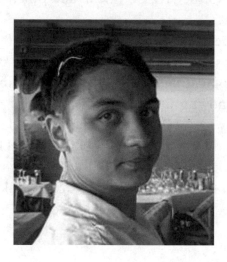

I am the older son, grandson and nephew in a family that has Hunting-ton's. I am happily married, studying at university and live in West London. I love playing guitar and football (though I play less and watch more nowadays) and going to see live bands. I'm not from a 'normal' family as my mother and father divorced when I was very young. Luckily Mum remarried my second father (I have two – greedy, I know). My biological father lives in Brunei, a small country on the island of Borneo.

Well, that's my CV, so I hope I have the job, and this is my story, so far…

The beginning

I have no memory of suddenly finding out what HD was. I have a series of memories of picking up bits and pieces of information about it that seem to have led to the point I am at now. My first memories of the disease were going to see my granddad at his London flat. I was young, only about seven or eight. I didn't know him very well. A history of violence and alcoholism had forced him and my grandma apart when I was a baby. This, we later discovered, was due to HD.

The only discernible memories I have of that day were the over-powering smell of tobacco smoke, the nicotine-stained computer and Brian (my granddad) giving me all the change in a little wooden box he kept on the shelf. A sum total of probably six pounds; I was ecstatic. But not for long. It was obvious to me even then that he was unwell. He was using walking sticks at this time, as he was struggling to stay upright. I could only guess this was due to the disease. I hate seeing people struggling with the things that most take for granted, such as walking, so to see one of my family members in this state was horrific. I think that was the last time I saw him living on his own, as he was later moved to a nursing home.

The nursing home

When my mum used to say we were going to see Brian at the nursing home I would internally protest, but smile and agree. I hated the drive from London to the country. It took about two hours, and a stifling sadness always filled the car on the way. Once we arrived we would walk through a hospital-like area – through corridors connecting big rooms with people sitting around them – to Brian's room. That walk was always strange, passing people who had no idea where they were, or were just incapable of looking after themselves. I used to think to myself, 'My granddad's not like this, is he?' When we arrived at Brian's room, we would often take him outside into the garden. He was in a wheelchair by this time. The garden was beautiful, and overlooked rolling green fields, with horses often roaming freely in the background. The smell of flowers and cut grass was a stark contrast from the odour of decay inside the building.

Eventually (I think I was 14 or 15) Brian died. I wasn't entirely sure how to react. I didn't know him very well, and found it hard to be around him. I actually knew my great-grandfather (Maggie's dad, or my mum's mum's dad, that is) better than I knew Brian. My mum was obviously devastated at her dad's death and I felt guilty for not feeling the same way. When Mum told me he had died, I was in my bedroom with one of my friends, who asked me if I wanted him to go home. But I didn't feel any emotion, so I said no.

After the funeral, time passed and we all got on with our lives. Over the years I started noticing Mum's physical control slipping very gradually – things dropping out of her hands and her walking being a bit unbalanced, for example. I tried to ignore it, but as I knew what HD was by this time, I got worried. I even tried to convince myself that she was practising her crappy punk dancing around the house and that it wasn't involuntary movements. Sorry, Mum, I'm going to get a clip around the ear for that one.

This went on for a while, probably a couple of years, and I knew that if I had noticed, then my step-dad Phil would have too. He had. He pulled me aside one day and asked me if I thought Mum was OK. I was shocked, but I knew that this conversation was inevitable, and had a whole speech planned in my head about how I knew, and how we could deal with it. I could only answer with, 'Yeah, she seems fine to me.' It was too much for me to admit.

After that discussion we came to the conclusion that there was a 90 per cent chance that Mum had it. At this point Mum had said to Phil that she didn't want the test that would show if she had the Huntington's gene, because she didn't want to know. This posed a dilemma. If we knew and she didn't and didn't want to know, we would have to keep it to ourselves (confusing eh?). I really didn't like this dishonesty. Not only would we have to deal with HD in the family, but we would also have to keep it a secret.

School, education and work

To find out that you have HD in your family in your early teens is tough, a time when you should be having fun and/or concentrating on schoolwork turns into an internal battle with yourself. My 'A' level grades – the exams we take at the end of school in the UK – were bad, so bad that the smell of failure stuck with me for years after. I was taking two subjects. I dropped out of one, Design & Technology, and got a bad grade for the other, Art & Design, well below what I was capable of. I couldn't understand what was happening, as I had always been quite capable academically.

This downward spiral carried on into my working life. After finishing my 'A' levels I decided to get a traineeship in IT. I got one, and with a good company to boot, making racing cars of all things. It was a teenage boy's dream first job. 'What do you do?' 'Work for a company that makes Indy cars and Formula One cars.' I thought things were on the up. I had a girlfriend at the time, passed my driving test and took a loan out to get a car. I passed my traineeship ahead of schedule and got a pay rise.

Yet still I had something niggling away at me in the back of my head that I was choosing to ignore. Then things began to go awry. I lost my job, just as it seemed to be going really well. I walked out of it, in fact; literally just walked out one day and didn't go back. My relationship with my girlfriend of the time became mutually destructive, I couldn't afford to maintain my car or pay for petrol and eventually the fragile world I had built up around myself collapsed. I started to believe I was flawed somehow, incapable of succeeding in life.

I only retell these stories to emphasize the amount of damage suppressing your emotions with something like HD can do to you. I

chose to ignore it and hope it would go away. It didn't and mani-
fested itself in some of the most horrific moments of my life so far.
Although I don't regret it, as I've learnt much from going through
these experiences, I would strongly recommend taking steps to
avoid such problems yourself.

Confidence and lack of it

There is one thing in me that really has been affected throughout
my entire HD experience. It's my confidence. HD seemed to suck it
right out of me, particularly at the low point described above. Prior
to us discovering HD was in the family, I was quite an outgoing,
friendly and, more often than not, noisy person. When HD reared
its ugly head, I shrivelled like crisp packets used to do if you put
them in the oven (that's 'chip' packets to Americans). The English
packets used to shrivel if you put them in the oven, with the writing
on them shrinking, too, to make perfectly formed miniature plastic
versions of the original that you could wear like a badge. Yes, I had
an experimental childhood.

I became alternately aggressive and extremely shy. I was in my
late teens at the time, so hormones would not have helped much.
Once I realized how low my self-esteem and confidence had gone, I
took steps to try and improve them. I read a lot of those self-
improvement books designed to develop your sense of self. I still
find them useful, actually. And I decided to go back to where I felt I
had failed – my education – and prove to myself that I could do it.
That's why I am in the middle of a degree now. I find that dealing
with HD is a lot easier when you notice the effects it is having on
your confidence and do something about it to fight back.

One of the most useful motivational quotes I came across in my
reading up on self-esteem and confidence is stuck on my wall. It's
the Henry Ford quote: 'If you think you can, or think you can't,
you're probably right.' It's something I would recommend to
anyone who has HD in their family. I mean, take stock and analyse

your mental state for areas of your life that Huntington's might be affecting without you realizing it. You often don't become aware of how badly something like this affects you, particularly the way it can sap your confidence and make you feel blighted, as if you are different from other people and can't succeed in their world any more because the HD won't let you. These feelings are often something you are just not consciously aware of until you step back and chart the progress of your life from how you were before you knew HD was in the family (if you didn't know at some stage, that is), through your initial discovery to the point you are at now.

After sitting back and analysing certain pivotal moments in my life where things seemed to have gone into a downward spiral, I realized that most of the major disruptions, where the course of my life became particularly bumpy, were due to my reaction to Huntington's. At the time my mum, grandma and step-father all recommended that I go and see a counsellor; I could see no reason for this as I felt my life was fine. Listen to your family. I didn't and it really made my formative years difficult. I was a teenage guy who wanted to go out, be macho and have a laugh with my friends. The last thing I wanted to do was to see a counsellor.

The day we were sure

More time passed (as it does) and Mum seemed to have come to the conclusion that she might have the illness herself. She took the test. She had HD. Oh crap. I don't remember much about this period of my life. Just as well probably. I can't remember who told me, whether it was Mum or Phil. I just remember a feeling of 'Oh, well, we knew that anyway.' As the disease is slow in the changes it brings to the affected person, it didn't seem an immediate threat. Mum didn't change as far as I could tell. She was still the embarrassing punk rocker she had always been (sorry, Mum) and still as outgoing and passionate as ever. I can only imagine the internal battle of torment and horror she must have been going through in admitting to herself that she had the disease.

I do, however, remember that on the day we found out for sure, I was working at a local pub. I decided after I had found out that Mum had the gene that I was fine and went into work as usual that day. I worked for a couple of hours and everything was great. I started talking to one of the bar workers and the conversation got on to how she had crashed her mum's car into their garage wall and scratched all the paintwork. She kept going on about how her mum would do this and that when she found out. On and on it seemed to go. I walked out of the pub; I couldn't bear to hear her pointless ranting about her scratched car. 'Come and live a day in my shoes,' I felt like saying. I didn't though.

This is an easy trap to fall into. Back then I found that everyone else's problems paled in comparison to mine. I had it the hardest, and nobody else's came even close. I'm not sure if this was a defensive mechanism or if my teenage hormones were playing with me again, but it is not a good way to live. There is always someone worse off than you, no matter how bad you ever think it gets.

The Look of Doom!

There are certain things that really get to me about Huntington's. One that used to hit me quite hard was people staring. Sometimes when we used to go out with Mum I would catch someone staring, laughing or pointing. I used to get very angry and want to cause them some physical pain. I was never brave or stupid enough to do this. So I developed something I named The Look of Doom™. Whenever I noticed someone staring, I would shoot a look in their direction, staring back at *them* in such a manic way that they would immediately know that it was not OK to continue what they were doing. Ninety-nine per cent of the time it worked.

The one time it didn't was when a rather burly figure of a man took it as a challenge to his masculinity and started shouting and advancing menacingly towards me. I looked away, steered Mum hastily in a different direction and he lost interest. I have now retired 'The Look of Doom' on safety grounds. Instead, I tend to feel sorry for the people who point and stare. To be as unaware of the fact that Mum obviously is unwell as these people are, is an ongoing mystery to me. I pity their ignorance.

Anyway, life has its ups and downs, and inevitably goes on. Mum's symptoms are obviously worse now than they used to be. It's the best part of a decade since we found out for sure that she has the illness. As HD affects your motor skills and nervous system, walking is much harder for her now. She has to eat a high-calorie diet to replace all the energy lost from the involuntary movements she constantly has. There are no complaints from her over this though.

Friendship and laughter

She is no longer able to drive, which threatened to isolate her even more for a while, till she managed to get some alternatives in place – organized support to take her out. She rarely sees her friends. I think that this is due to one or two of them being scared of HD and what it has done to Mum. She has close friends who are not too far away who you might expect to be rallying around her, but who seem to find it too painful and haven't adapted by learning how to chat with her now. Well, if that's the case, then imagine how she feels.

Still, she has some brilliant new friends, like Jo from The Clive Project, who have come into her life specifically because of HD. And among her old friends there are some amazing ones. Mum has one friend who lives almost at the tip of Scotland, hundreds of miles away from us. Helen has known Mum since they were both small children. To see Helen and her husband, children and parents with Mum – Phil took her up to stay with them for a few days a while ago and told me about this – is a true lesson in what friendship is. They are incredibly attentive, unfazed by how she has changed, and they laugh with her. Mum's sense of humour is completely un-dimmed, and all she needs is for people to listen and give her half a second to get her one-liners out and anyone who has known her would realize that she is as sharp and sarcastic as ever.

As a family, we still know how to laugh, too. The jokes are usually at each others' expense. And Mum still keeps us all in check, usually with a slap on the back or a cushion to the head. It has to be said that Huntington's can be very funny, in a slapstick kind of way. And you should laugh at it. One particular memory that sticks in my mind is an incident that my brother doesn't even remember, and probably for good reason. We had all just walked into the living room, having come in from a day out. Danny, my brother, was standing by the main light switch on the wall. I was standing in front of him talking to Mum. Before I go on, you have to understand Mum has a tendency to unexpectedly jerk forwards or backwards and head-butt innocent bystanders, not on purpose (at least I think not), but due to HD.

So I was unexpectedly head-butted. As a reflex, my head shot back into my brother's head. His head then flew back and hit the light switch. The lights went out. We stood in the darkness, shocked at what had happened, with at least two of us nursing a bumped head and wondering if everything going black meant concussion had set in. Mum was first to break the silence. 'Why did you turn the lights out, I was talking to you?' she said, mystified.

Super strength

There are many symptoms associated with HD. One that I don't think has yet been identified is that of superhuman strength. Since Mum's initial discovery that she has HD her physical power has increased until it now seems to match the Incredible Hulk. When we visit my parents I am shocked at the catalogue of sheer destruction that has happened since the last time we were there. Towel rails have been pulled off the wall, kitchen cupboard handles are ripped off, toilet seats smashed, there are splatters of ketchup on the ceiling (yes, ketchup). The list is endless.

It also gets quite frustrating coming to visit only to be met with a list of things that need fixing, as my wife and I are often the ones doing the running repair work that Phil can't deal with. This is basically everything beyond tightening a screw. His do-it-yourself skills have always been noticeable by their absence. Unfortunately, Chan and I are quite good at it.

As well as being funny (how did that ketchup get up there?), the capacity for destruction can be awe inspiring. The towel rail that parted company from the wall, for example, happened in a bathroom Chantel and I had recently redecorated. During our redecoration we had tried to remove the rail. It was stuck fast to the wall, we could not budge it. So we painted around it. But, along comes Mum a month or two later and, presumably drying her hands, rips the thing off the wall. Oh, to have the strength of my mother.

Family ties

Which reminds me of that old story about sticks. Maybe you know it. One stick on its own can be snapped quite easily. Get a little bundle of sticks together and you find you can't snap them. It represents the power of family. Geddit? Discovering HD is in the family, it's more important than ever to stick together ('Stick together?'– sorry about that). I think nowadays that the majority of the time we do stick together. It wasn't always that way, though. There was an initial period where we all kept to ourselves and dealt with it all internally. This, I feel, pulled the family apart. This is no longer the case, as we all work together for the greater good. Actually, that's true of our nuclear family. But, if you step back a bit and look at the bigger family, there are members who have clashed with each other over Huntington's and haven't spoken for a couple of years. We're hoping this will change.

My wife

Talking of family strength brings me to my wonderful wife. When I first met Chantel I was at a low point in my life. I would use drinking and clubbing with my friends as an escapist's route to a happier life. It didn't actually make me feel any better, but it did let me forget for the four or five hours I would be out. And as fate would have it, I met my lovely wife-to-be on one of these booze fuelled nights.

When I initially told her of the disease I was scared how she would react. I didn't want to admit to her that I had a weakness (which is how it seemed, that I was revealing a secret weakness), but felt an honest approach was the only way to go. If we were to become a long-term couple, then she would undoubtedly find out anyway. She reacted astonishingly well, due to the fact that she had studied the disease at school (fate, methinks).

We have had, since then, many discussions about HD, mainly consisting of me ranting and raving about how crap the whole situation is. And always she listens, nods her head and tells me if I'm being a plonker (if you're not in the UK, that's a hard word to translate). She has been a guiding light when things seemed dark for me, and I think that I might still be where I was emotionally five years ago if not for her.

The one thing that really helped turn my life around was to have someone to talk to. I found it hard to talk to my family about HD, as they all had their own problems and issues to deal with at the time. My wife has an objective point of view and would be brutally honest if I had said something that was selfish or in any way self-indulgent. Having someone like this is precious, as you know you can trust them.

My mother...and memories

I have always loved and admired my mum, mainly for her strong will, loving nature and her 'I don't care what other people think' attitude. When I was growing up, we were a close-knit family unit of Mum, my step-dad, myself and later my little brother. We always did everything together. Family holidays would usually involve great nights out where we would all get dressed up to the nines and stay up really late. Getting ready to go out was half the fun. Mum would always dance around the room before any excursion, much to my brother's (and my) embarrassment.

Mum and I have always been close, probably due to the fact that when my biological dad left we were on our own for a while. It's very difficult to watch as someone you love is gradually taken away from you. That's what Huntington's does, gradually moves the person you love further and further away from you, as if you are watching a very slow train recede into the distance. In my opinion, the gradual nature of it is the worst part of it all. It's happened over so many years that it almost seems that Mum has always been that way. It's hard to remember the 'good old days'. But we discovered a cache of old family videos recently, which brought the memories flooding back and made us all smile.

Mum always used to put together photo albums after each of our holidays, one album for each trip. And Phil has taken to putting old family holiday pictures up on every available square inch of wall surface. As you walk around the house, you are confronted by our happy, smiling faces at various ages. The most recent ones have my wife Chan in too, so walking down the corridor in our house is like walking through time, taking a trip through our family history. I realized recently he put them up on purpose as a constant reminder of the happy times we have had as a family.

The photographic album record has fizzled out, as it's not something Mum can organize for herself any more. Maintaining your family memories is a vital part of reminding us all of what we are part of. So, when we were living at their house recently, Chan spent an afternoon with Mum going through old photos – everything from Mum's childhood to our wedding – and, where Chan didn't know, asking who all the people were in the pictures. Chan made notes and then put the pictures into albums and wrote next to each picture who everybody was.

'Memories are self-defining and support our identity', I read somewhere a while ago. When something like Huntington's is chipping away at your identity, the more reinforcements you are surrounded with, the better. The photos on the walls, the old family videos and the photo albums are like having a series of defences built around yourself.

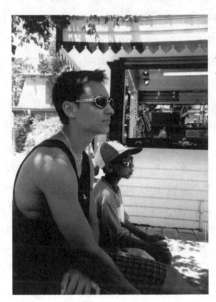

Twins separated by ten years. Me, 17. Dan, 7, checking out the talent, Key West, Florida. Dan's saying, 'I don't like the look of yours.'

My 'twin' brother

There is a ten year age gap between my brother and myself. And we have different fathers. Despite that, as we were growing up, everyone said we were twins separated by ten years. Old friends of the family who came to visit would shout, 'My God! You have another Bromley all over again. He's Bromley's twin!' By the time Danny was two he had heard this so many times that he believed it. We were on holiday in the Lake District and Phil and I were out on the lake on a rented boat while Mum and Dan were in the tearoom waiting for us, as it was too cold and wet for them (wimps). A friendly old lady started chatting to Dan, Mum told us later, and said, 'And do you have any brothers or sisters?' Danny piped up, 'Yes, I've got one twin brother, but he's twelve and I'm two.'

Despite our age difference we have always got on very well and been very close. When he was born it was like I had a new toy. Until I had to start changing nappies, that is. As with any relationship between brothers, the older feels responsible for making sure the younger is safe and happy. That's particularly so when you are twins separated by ten years. But, the one thing that really threatens either and both of us is the one thing I can do nothing about.

Having moved away to London to start my university course, I feel a guilt that can only be described as having abandoned my family. I feel this most for my brother, as he is at the age I was when things got tough for me. I really want to be there for him, but I know I would be doing the rest of my family no favours by staying at home and not making something of myself. So I chose to take the lesser of two evils.

My step-dad

I can split our relationship into three parts, pre-HD, HD part 1 and HD part 2. Pre-HD we were very close and he was everything you could wish for from a step-father. I never really saw him as a step-father as we were a very close family unit and he and my mum had got together when I was very young. We laughed and joked and he always treated me like his own son.

HD part 1 was a difficult time for all of us and the strain it put on the relationship between us was immense. We gradually lost touch with our old relationship and formed a new one that wasn't healthy for either of us. As we both dealt with HD in different ways, a clash of personalities ensued. This went on for a while until I finally left home.

HD part 2 is the stage we're at now. We have both come to terms with the emotional barrage that HD fires at you and have rebuilt our relationship. We get along really well now and are always helping each other out. This makes our HD ordeal easier for us and the whole family.

My grandmother

I don't think that I would be where I am today without the love and support of my grandmother, Maggie. We have always been very close. She is someone who can light up the room with a single cackle of laughter, and a person I would always go out of my way to please. Having been through an extremely difficult HD break-up herself, she has come out the other side laughing, smiling and still believing there is good in the world. That is an inspiration to me. When my home life was difficult she would always be there and tell me if I was being a prat.

One of the most admirable aspects of my grandmother is how she deals with HD. Having lived through a tough break-up due to HD, and then finding out that two of her three children have it, which in turn puts all of her grandchildren via those two children at risk, and yet to still smile and bustle around looking after everyone, is amazing. I often use her as an inspiration when things get tough. I think she's like the beating heart of our family sometimes. Chantel did a week's work experience at the library Maggie worked in until recently, and said whatever room Maggie was in at any given moment would turn into the centre of laughter for the whole building. She's infectious.

Friends

Friends come and go. I guess from their point of view, I come and go, too, particularly as we (Chan and I) have moved around the country and even across to the other side of the world and back over the past few years. It is only when you have to deal with something potentially life altering like HD in your family that you find out who your true friends really are. I've lost touch with many friends, but the ones I am still in touch with are really my strength. My best friend is a mad Canadian musician who can talk about anything and everything to anybody and always makes me laugh when all feels lost. When I met him outside a train station in London recently after not seeing him for a few months, he ran towards me, with a rucksack and guitar on his back and jumped on me with one of his Canadian bear hugs. I ended up flat on my back on the street, with a Canadian, a rucksack and a guitar on top of me, looking rather odd, as he wouldn't let go.

He has been there for me through thick and thin, and is always in my corner. When he first found out about HD and met my mum for the first time, he didn't bat an eyelid. He smiled, cracked two beers open, one for her and one for himself and proceeded to have a conversation about god knows what into the early hours of the morning.

Testing times

People often ask me why I haven't had the test myself, the one that tells you if you have the Huntington's gene or not. This is a bit of a bone of contention for me. I can only reply that I don't think that having the test would improve my life in any way, no matter what the result. If I don't have it, then great, but that still leaves my brother and my uncle's children at risk. It's that old 'all in the same boat' thing. I'd feel as if I'd been airlifted out of the boat, shouting, 'I'm fine, so I'm going. See ya,' leaving them bobbing about in stormy waters on their own. That sounds a bit melodramatic, but I'm sure you get what I mean.

If I do have the gene then I would have to live my life wondering when the symptoms of the disease were going to start. If this was the case then how would I ever achieve anything in my life? No I don't want to know now, as eventually I will anyway. If someone else's life depended on it then I would want to know. But the only circumstance I can foresee as warranting my testing would be if children were involved.

Children

My wife and I have discussed whether to have children on several occasions. This is a big issue for people at risk of Huntington's. In fact, one of the first things my mum was told when she discovered she was at risk of inheriting it was a matter-of-fact 'Oh, we advise people in your situation not to have children.' This was delivered by a particularly cold consultant, in an off-hand way. Mum says the message she received from that was 'We don't want the risk of any more of your kind around if we can help it.'

But, when Chan and I discuss kids, it's not in those terms. It's in the same terms every other couple discuss what their children might be like. 'I bet it would have your nose,' says my wife. 'Poor thing!' I reply. It's not the right time for us to have children at the moment, but eventually we will. The patter of tiny feet would be a blessing, and any child hallowed with the conk that is my nose will be a sight to see.

We still have a lot of things to do with our life before we have children. So we will cross that bridge when we come to it. We know there are options. Chan writes about that in her chapter.

It's getting better…man

OK, so up until this point my contribution to this family book has all been pretty heavy. I did this on purpose and apologize for any boxes of tissues I may have caused you to work your way through if you collapsed in floods of tears. I spent time on the difficult stuff with good reason though, partly because there is at times only tough stuff to deal with when Huntington's is the subject. But also

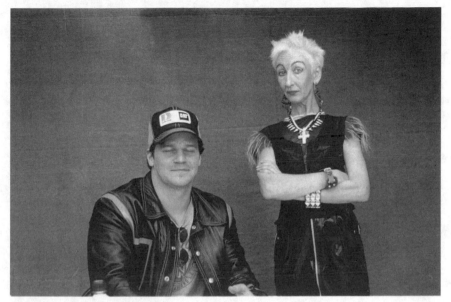

Mum meets her idol, David Boreanaz, who plays Angel in the TV series *Buffy The Vampire Slayer* and *Angel*. He was so overwhelmed by Mum's fashion sense he had to close his eyes.

because we are all fans of the TV show *Angel* in our family. That's a spin-off series from *Buffy The Vampire Slayer*, for those who don't know. We are not necessarily fans by choice, more by the indoctrination that comes with constant exposure.

You see, Mum fancies the pants off David Boreanaz, who plays the lead character in the series, and watches it on DVD over and over again. When she's not watching the DVDs, she watches the endless repeats on TV. So we all end up watching it. Phil even took her to meet him once at a fan convention. Anyway, the creator of *Angel* and *Buffy* talks a lot about 'the arc' of the story, how a story has to start in one place, achieve a trajectory and end up somewhere it has been aiming for.

We all (the family members) discussed this before writing our chapters and concluded that our arc was that the first few years of finding out HD is in the family are absolute sh*t. But that the challenge is then to create a curve of your own as a family in which you are getting stronger and putting extra support in place from each other, friends, family, outside agencies, that matches the arc that is prescribed by the symptoms of the disease getting worse. If you can keep ahead of it, making yourself stronger and supporting the other members of the family, then you don't feel quite so out of control.

Now for the good stuff

My life turned around when I finally realized that worrying would get me nowhere. This epiphany changed my perception of HD completely. Yes it's a horrible experience to see someone having to deal with something like Huntington's, especially a family member. But no matter how much you worry about it, it won't get any better. So don't waste your energy on all the anxiety and worry. I'm not saying that not worrying about it makes it all go away, but it takes your focus off what is wrong with the world and places it on what you can do to make the world better.

Chan and I bought Phil a little plaque as a birthday present a while ago, as he used to be the biggest worrier on the planet. It says on it 'Worry is like a rocking chair, keeps you busy, but never gets you anywhere.' Cheesy but true.

I'm older, wiser and probably uglier now. I've learnt many things when trying to deal with this hereditary disease. The one thing I always found hard was that I couldn't fight it if I got it. There is no way for me to physically or mentally beat it. Frustration was a major part of my life as a result. I tended to disappear into myself to escape what was really happening. I felt I was in a constant battle with myself to keep my head above water some days. Other days were great, days when you almost forget about HD, when it gets pushed into the background of your life.

To counter the bad days when Huntington's worries look as if they are about to creep up and swarm all over me, I've developed a couple of mental word tricks that come in useful. Like The Look of Doom™ (see above), I've trademarked these techniques, so if you need to use them for yourself contact me to discuss the royalty fee.

(For American readers, that is what we Brits call irony, by the way. Or straightforward British sarcasm if you prefer.)

One of my techniques owes a little to Monty Python. It is a bit like a Zen state of mind. I call it 'The Attitude of Meh' ('Meh' pronounced a bit like 'Ni', as in 'The Knights Who Say "Ni"' in one of the Monty Python films). 'Meh' is what I say to myself when things are getting on top of me. Using 'Meh, it's all right' or 'Meh, it doesn't matter' is enough to turn the tide of a day for me. Powerful stuff. You read it here first.

'Hunting Don' is another way I like to think of it. If you can shrink the thing you fear and turn it into something laughable, you shrink the fear itself. So I think of a silly little man named Don, who wanders around taunting people yet always, somehow, eludes capture. Well, we're hunting you, my family, other families, doctors, carers and a whole host of scientists with drooling, angry bloodhounds. By giving this illness a personality (and a rather bad one at that) then I can take the sting out of its tail and beat it mentally.

I'm also lucky to have a great family. I love them all very much and probably wouldn't be here today without their support and love. Literally. And although I do tend to worry occasionally about my brother, mum and step-dad, I know that they have the support of my grandmother who lives nearby. I also go to Oxfordshire with my wife as often as I can, as it's only an hour or so's drive from where we live. And we all go on holiday together once a year, with me eating too much, my brother half-drowning in the pool (or at least he used to – he's learnt to swim now unfortunately), my step-dad gracing us with the annual spectacle of his hairy legs, and my wife and mum trying to turn brown but turning bright pink instead.

Found again

Other members of the family, particularly my parents, say that they feel they lost me for a few years as I struggled to come to terms with

Huntington's, but that now I've found myself again. I am a changed man. I decided to go to university (and got in!) and have many side projects running as well, from designing websites for people to starting a record label with my Canadian musician friend. I want to be successful in my life now and believe I will be. OK, so it's not easy continuing to live with HD in the family and there are obviously still plenty of bad days. You can't do anything about the bad things that HD throws at you. But you *are* responsible for how you react to them – the worry, stress and anger that make life such hard work – and *can* do something about those reactions.

If you're at risk, live your life well and to the full for the person or people in your family who have the illness already. It's important to cultivate within yourself the belief that whatever life, or Huntington's, throws at you next, you will be able to deal with it. In the immortal words of the *Eels* song 'Novocaine for the Soul', 'Life is hard, but so am I.'

CHAPTER 4

'Is Everyone All Right?'
The Younger Son's Story

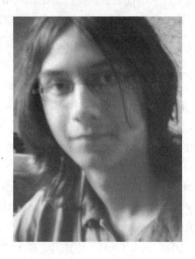

Describing yourself is always hard to do. But since you and I have never met and I am at the moment just text on a page to you, it is best that I tell you a little about me first. My name is Danny. Good start; got my name down. I am 15 years old, and already taller than my older brother and dad, much to their annoyance. I'm skinny, rather tanned thanks to my Indian granddad's family, and have long black hair, which desperately needs a trim. Not a lot else I can say about myself physically. I could go on about my shoe size for another few pages if you like, but I'm guessing the majority of sane people out there would prefer I change the subject.

I think I'm size eight and a half by the way.

As I'm sure you've already guessed I hate describing myself. Say certain things and you come across as a big-head, whilst others just make you seem completely idiotic or that you are faking modesty. When I asked Dad for some words to sum me up, he said I used to go around asking everyone if they were all right, like it was my job to check the family was OK. That's why Mum titled this chapter 'Is everyone all right?' Thanks. I won't be saying that again, then.

I thought I'd duck out of any more self-description completely and instead ask people who know me to describe me to you (still with me?). Warning: it's a biased version of me, since they're my friends, so don't believe any of it for a second. Here goes…

Me, according to some friends

> Chris: You are fun to be around because you are always up for a laugh, you tend to take a leading role within our group, you are possibly the most moral person I know, which is good because that makes you one of the most loyal people I know, but is sometimes bad because you get slightly too bothered about other people's business (like people drinking). Probably your best quality is that you're willing to make friends with anyone who deserves it, you don't care what idiots from the 'cool' crowd think, which is a wicked thing because frankly I doubt your shenanigans[1] have made you the most popular guy in the year, but more importantly you're always there for those who matter.

> Abbi: You are very caring and you care about other people a lot which can be a bad thing at times as you don't care about yourself enough. I think you worry a

---

1   Danny has a tendency to take on anyone he feels is being unfair or bullying others, and very loudly tells them where they are going wrong. This has earned him a bit of a reputation as mouthy at school. And we're proud of him for it.

bit too much about others sometimes and not yourself. You work hard and you like writing which I think you are very good at, and you're not really a sporty person. I think you are very funny and witty and a positive person with a positive attitude. I don't think you are very sociable but under the circumstances that is completely understandable.

Becky: When I think about Danny I think:

1. You're very private; don't always know when to tell people what's wrong in your life.

2. You try to deal with things on your own because you don't like to worry others.

3. You don't think you're as special as everyone else when really you are.

4. You have to be the funniest guy I know and most carefree (you never let little things get you down).

5. You can be pig-headed.

6. But saying that, when you're in the wrong you always make up for it by being so apologetic.

7. You're always sensitive when talking about people. People know what you say is what you truly mean.

8. You're a brilliant friend; somebody I can trust not to just be there when I need but to tell me when I need to be realistic.

I was cringing as I read that myself. I can imagine you all thinking what a big-head I am! Thank you so much to all three of those friends for finding it in your time to do this, and for your friendship in general. Your payment is a place in this book and my heart. (Yeah, other friends, you're in my heart too, but I've been told to keep the word count down here.)

This is normal

My role in the family is, in general, to be the younger sibling: clumsy, barely know how to cook or clean, and tend to stand in the background making sarcastic comments at everyone else. It's the lowest form of wit, I know, so just right for me. If I go too far I know Brom (older brother) will just pick me up over his shoulder and launch me across the room, meaning I tend to avoid making a complete nuisance of myself.

Other than that my life revolves around school, video games, friends, family and the computer. As already mentioned in one of the quotes above, I'm not very sociable and have become infamous amongst my gang of mates for never finding the time to go out and have fun with them. Mainly because, in all honesty, I'm a lazy sod. I blame my teenage hormones. Always.

Being the youngest, I think it was probably easiest for me to adapt to this way of life – I mean growing up with Huntington's in the family and seeing its effects – because it's all I've known, in a way.

It hasn't made me bitter and twisted. I mean I don't envy other people for having a healthy family or anything like that. I have accepted it as part of my life, since there really is nothing else that I can do. I can't complain, argue, or make it go away as that's not how these things work. I was still growing up when I found out so I absorbed the information more easily, I think. My brother was a lot older at the time and just maturing. It hit him a lot harder, as he was reaching adulthood, when having to rethink your whole life can be a lot harder.

Dad tells me that according to research the younger you are when you find out, the easier it is. Because you don't form a sense of what is normal life and then have that snatched away from you. It (living with the HD) just kind of *is* your normal life right from the start.

Just another teen

One plus point of being a teenager having to deal with HD is that I'm not the only one with a 'problem' at my age: I never see myself as worse off than anyone in my own year group, because *every* teenager nowadays (probably as in every recent generation) knows they have more problems in their life than anyone else. So, if others see me as a teenager with a problem because I have HD in my family, then I'm in good company because we've all got problems.

In a surprising number of cases, in my experience, my peers are coping with some very serious stuff which, to them, is a mountain of a problem that won't go away. When weighing my problems up against others', mine may sometimes look bigger and more horrible to some people, but I'm lucky in that I never look at it like that. Basically, everyone's got troubles and no matter how big or small they look from the outside, it's how big they are to you that counts.

The white water ride

So, the starting point for me is that Huntington's gives you an accepting outlook on life when you've known about it for ages and haven't had an existing sense of 'normal' destroyed by it. That is probably why I am able to write about this disease that has come crashing down on my family without the writing being too difficult or painful, as I think it is for other members of my family contributing to this book, judging by the stressy looks I see on their faces when I know they've been writing their chapter.

In short, this illness has destroyed a lot of my mother's freedom and taken away her future. In the process, it has taken the rest of us out of the calm, shallow waters most people seem to live in and into a kind of emotional white water ride. So my clothes get a bit wet now and again as we try and navigate our way through the emotional rapids that HD tends to put families through. I can hardly complain when I see other people facing the same situation without giving up or going under. Instead of seeing no hope for us (as some people might do from the outside if they are told about the cold, hard facts of the illness and how it progresses) I actually marvel at the strength of the people around me.

My father and Chan, my sister-in-law, have both had many an opportunity to swim off and find a more peaceful life away from the emotional rapids that HD drags you over. Still they throw themselves in regardless. They didn't have to. In many families, the husband or wife of a person with Huntington's makes a run for it. They're just too scared to face it and they escape to try and make a normal life elsewhere.

Brom, my brother, has never stopped giving me morale boosts and little words of comfort and support (in between punches on the arm and dead legs), pulling me up whenever he senses I may be slipping under the water, even if only for a second – basically looking out for his little brother. And Mum is a true beacon of encouragement, still finding that glimmer of light inside her that pushes her ever onwards and up. She still gets up and greets the day with a noisy 'Good morning!' yelled at everyone enthusiastically.

None of us has lost sight of the fact that life is there to be enjoyed. In fact, if anything, we enjoy it more.

Friendship

Each member of my family has set an example for me and I refuse to allow myself to become a moody teenager when they're making such an effort. It's not a conscious decision, more a survival instinct as Dad once put it; kicking in as the Huntington's Disease symptoms progress and not allowing me to fall down and weep.

So my outstanding family has kept me going but I must not forget that, at my age, friendship is another major factor that keeps you sane. I won't mention any more names because I don't want to invade their privacy, but there are people out there, across the world even, if you include my internet friends, who have been awe-inspir-ingly helpful and supportive.

If you might be in a similar situation to me – in a family where there is some ongoing serious problem like a critical illness – and there's only one piece of information you take away from my blather, it is this: do not lose sight of your friends. Let them know how much you appreciate them, surprise them with little thoughtful gifts, and listen when they need to speak. In return you will be able to share your time with the most amazing people around, and you'll know that there are people out there caring for you. There will be a few days in your life when you'll be gob-smacked by just how far your friends will go for you, so never forget how important they are.

None of them paid me for that paragraph. I'll have to chase them up for the cash.

My history of events

I guess the wise thing to do now would be a small history of events. It's difficult for me to recall the first time I ever learnt about HD, since I can barely remember what I did last week. There was never really an 'announcement' of sorts. If there was I don't seem to be able to recall it at all.

Possibly the main turning point was back when I was ten, just after school. As per usual I walked in and prepared to throw myself on the sofa when I realized we had guests sitting on it already. I'm not sure how reliable my brain is on this subject, but I recall two women, sitting opposite my parents. As soon as I arrived, Dad steered me into the kitchen and put the kettle on. Minutes later I was sipping my tea (typical of us English folk) and listened as my dad explained all – the full nature of the illness and the implications for me and my brother in terms of chances of inheriting it.

That was the first time I took Huntington's Disease seriously as part of our lives. On one level I must have known about it well before then. But, I can't say I remember my granddad in the nursing home when I was small. And he died when I was five. The illness in the family was something I knew about but didn't really pay much attention to. Anyway, apparently, the two women visitors were a social worker who specialized in genetic illnesses and Carol, our local support worker from the Huntington's Disease Association.

Dad went on to tell me how Mum had taken the test to see if she had the gene that her dad died of and that it had come back positive. I think they all said I shouldn't worry that she would suddenly die or anything like that – that this thing took decades and was gradual.

I can't remember exactly how I took it. I'd always known my mum was 'different'; unconventional, if you like. After all, most parents don't stand in the school playground to pick you up decked out with spiked hair and a leather jacket. But finding out that wasn't the only thing about her that was different was still a moment which makes the heart seem to stop, the stomach churn. No matter how cushioned you are, or how much you prepare yourself by having been told about the possibilities, you are never ready to learn that your parent has a terminal illness.

Afterwards I sat in the living room, next to my parents, facing the people telling us about our future. I managed to stay for at least an hour, but eventually when the conversation switched to something I couldn't understand, I headed for my room and shut the door. Since most of this memory is vague and clouded, I'm not sure if I broke down in tears or not. I do know, however, that I felt completely useless. I stood in the centre of the room, trying to think of something, anything I could do.

I never did find anything I could do. I flicked upstairs and downstairs during the next hour or so that they were discussing it, hardly listening to a word that was said in case it was something I could not bear. To be honest I'd never looked twice at my mum or thought anything other than that she was hyper-trendy. The punk hairdo, spiky bracelets, all just seemed part of her unique style. And as far as the movements went, I must have been blind since I had not really noticed them as being unusual before that occasion. Jangly bracelets just used to announce Mum's arrival in a room as a matter of course. Of course the movements caused the jangling: everything was now staring me in the face.

The social worker gave me her card before they left and told me to call her any time I might be worried about something or needed any advice about the illness or anything. I was ten years old, not a lot of chance of that happening. Almost like walking outside and unloading my problems to the first person on the street. What I mean is, I didn't know her well enough to want to tell her all my problems. I got another card recently, which I have been tempted to call once, but I'm not brave enough to pick up the phone.

Life goes on

After that day I carried on as if everything was normal. I wasn't about to become a depressive teenager prematurely at ten. As far as I was concerned, it would be 20 years more before the absolute worst happened to my mum – well, possibly. And even longer than that before I had to worry about my brother and then me maybe getting it, as the illness doesn't emerge till maybe your late thirties. At my age, that seemed like an awfully long way away. Still does I suppose.

I was probably brought up a lot better than I ever realized; or at least, that's the conclusion I have come to today. I must have had a few warning signs strategically placed before me and information planted at a young age to prepare me for the possible worst. And it must have subconsciously sunk in. Of course I can't remember any events offhand but I must have been prepared or else I would have taken it a lot worse.

I think that accounts for the years between the ages of five and ten when, if someone had said, 'What did your granddad die of?' I would probably have said, 'Can't remember. Er, Huntington's or something I think it's called.' But I didn't connect that with a risk to my mum or my brother and me. Your brain sometimes doesn't choose to put two and two together until it has to. So I hadn't consciously worked out how that could affect us later.

As the days went by after I was officially told that my mum had the same gene that killed my granddad, and that I had a 50 per cent chance of getting it when I grew up (as did my brother), it seemed to blend into my background more. I told neither teacher nor student about my mother's condition except when it was unavoidable. It was hardly that I did not want to say. Heck, everyone enjoys a little sympathy now and then. I just did not need to. If there were any problems going on within the family as a result of this news, they were shielded from me because I was quite young and blissfully unaware; something that I am grateful for.

To test or not to test

According to the facts I've managed to pick up, to be able to take the HD test I'll have to be 18. That's pretty obvious since most blood tests and the like require you to be 'of age', fully responsible and able to take whatever information is discovered by the test. It's also best to be in a calm period of your life; there'll be counselling, various visits to the centre over a month, everything to get you in the mental state. Preparing you for the worst, basically, or at least for the stress and nerves.

As far as I can tell, the testing process consists of: genetic counselling, a neurological exam, a psychological interview, a discussion of what the results could be and so on, then the blood test itself. They take you through the whole procedure by the hand. It never ceases to amaze me how much effort is put into all of it, how the people care for you and are always attempting to help you cope with the outcome. The doctors, nurses, psychiatrists, etc. who devote their time to people facing these scary tests are pretty impressive if you ask me.

I have yet to actually ask what happened when my mum took her test, though I know it would not be the same as mine. Hers was a confirmatory test, where they check the symptoms to see if the person actually *has* HD. She took a blood test later just to make 100 per cent sure, apparently. It came out the same.

The blood test is what definitely tells you, no doubt, if you have the gene or not. Personally, I'm not going to have fun with that needle, like most people, as I only have two injections in my memory so far; neither of them pleasant. The test I will be up for is a 'presymptomatic test', meaning checking the chromosomes to discover if the HD gene is in there or not. I had to mouth 'presymptomatic' quite a few times before I managed to write it down. Even Microsoft Word doesn't seem to recognize it.

I hardly need to say it, but I'm not looking forward to my eighteenth birthday. Fifty per cent, no matter how often I get told is perfectly evenly balanced as a probability, seems a lot larger than it should be; I mean the 50 per cent chance of having the rogue gene outweighs the 50 per cent chance of not having it – looms larger in my head, at least. My maths teacher would kill me for saying that as it makes no sense logically. However, I'm still definitely going to have the test, because I'm one of these people who need to know things. I'd be sick with worry not knowing. Whether it's bad or not, at least my mind will be put at rest and I won't be waking up in the middle of the night with the same question boring into my skull. I just have to know.[2]

---

2   The vast majority of people at risk of inheriting Huntington's Disease actually choose not to have the test that would confirm whether they have the HD gene or not. Often a young person is set on having the test as soon as they are old enough. But then, when they come of age, they choose to delay or postpone it, sometimes indefinitely. It seems to be about keeping options open: as long as you have decided not to take the test, you know that decision is always up for review. You can always change your mind; you have some control. But once the decision is made, the test taken, and the results discovered, there is no going back: there is no option to change your mind. You've walked through that door and there's no coming back.

Fears

My biggest fear at the moment is for my brother. He is getting on with his life, has already moved out of the house, got married and is halfway through his university education. Aged 25, he has just started to adjust to the life of an adult, though he still enjoys letting his hair down at any opportunity.

I can't help but feel that sometimes I am watching him from afar and crossing my fingers, because it would crush all of us if that life – all his plans and the things he is working towards – were to suddenly come to a standstill. I've always looked up to my brother, never thought that he could do better or ever let me down, and in no way would it be fair for him to inherit the disease. The trick is to carry on assuming that it won't happen. Otherwise it can paralyse you if you worry about the worst too much. 'Just get on with it' is a great approach to this thing. And Brom does.

Then again, I'm also absolutely petrified of getting it myself. Like I said I am clumsy, something which a lot of perfectly normal people are, but you can't help but pause when you drop that cup or stumble over that step.

I never have broken down in tears with the idea that I might have got it myself. But when you're caught unaware and find yourself unsure whether you permitted your body to make that move, or realize that you're talking too fast and people can't understand, it kicks in from behind and a panic can begin to rise. It takes a great deal of effort to jam it back into its cell, normally involving some form of yelling to scare the wits out of it and make sure it doesn't come back. I'm a bit of a melodramatic teenager, remember. Yelling is our answer to a lot of things.

The facts are there for me to face. There's a 50 per cent chance I'll get HD as an adult, which is lower than a lot of other hereditary diseases out there. Also there's a tiny percentage chance that anyone who inherits the disease will contract it at a really young age – 'Juvenile Onset HD' or something like that they call it; it's incredibly rare so there is no reason for me to worry. The fear just seems to be a knee-jerk reflex feeling that hits me when I am least prepared for it sometimes.

Effects on my life

Huntington's-related 'incidents', if I can put it like that, are going to start occurring more and more as the years go by. OK, by 'incidents' I mean sometimes Mum gets frustrated by the illness and slips into a temper which gets taken out on Dad, or she'll have the occasional heavy drinking episode, since people with Huntington's aren't good at regulating their intake and realizing when they have had enough. Mum loves drinking Jim Beam whiskey on a Friday night. She says she limits it to the weekend and explains that she has to have something to look forward to and that other people enjoy a drink so why shouldn't she. That is fair enough for her. If you have an illness that limits your life, then you have to be able to let your hair down and maybe forget it for a while, which I think the drink helps Mum to do.

But it's not a lot of fun for the people around her. I don't like being in the same room and so disappear upstairs to the computer or to my room a lot, as the effect of the drink seems to me to exaggerate the symptoms – dropping things and falling over and slurred speech – so I feel as if I am seeing her as she will be in a few years' time, when the illness has advanced further. It's upsetting so I keep out of her way most of the weekend. I'd like to be able to tell her that without hurting her feelings. Maybe this is a way of doing it.

One effect this has had on me is that I don't like seeing my friends drinking. It has stopped me from even trying any beer or wine, with the exception of a sip of champagne at very special occasions. To my friends this is startling; because no matter how sweet and naive adults would want to believe teenagers to be, they do enjoy a quick pint or two while no one is looking and wherever they can get it from.

The last time I saw one of my fellow teens clutching a can of beer I had to stop myself from shouting abuse at them about how stupid it was to drink, rather than smart and grown up. Luckily they didn't notice me scowling before I'd checked myself and walked off quickly. But I'm always pestering them all about drinking and they're always getting angry at me for constantly badgering them about it.

Apparently the drinking thing is linked to something called 'perseveration' in Huntington's Disease (as in 'persevere'). The person who has HD will often repeat the same things habitually, leading to chain-smoking (which Mum does) and, er, chain-drinking, I guess (which Mum also does). Having a drink is, for Mum, often a reaction to boredom and being stuck at home. She's a very independent person and loves having fun and going out, so it must be frustrating for her.

I also seem to have reacted strongly to the constant smoking in the house. I positively *hate* smoking. Whilst my friends can simply shrug when someone tells us about yet another teenager we know who thinks it's cool and has succumbed to the cancer-sticks, I over react. Once again this tracks back to my mum, as now she consumes about 50 each day without a second thought. If there aren't plenty more full packets in the cupboard (and she likes to check, for reassurance) she begins to get stressed.

I am very fortunate to have one or two friends who are very anti-smoking, providing me with back-up any time I need an outlet for having to live every day surrounded by something I hate so much. At the same time my more level-headed companions will give me a cuff around the ear and tell me to quieten down, which provides a good sense of balance – even if I have a sore ear for a while.

Keep getting stronger

We have the odd bad night. If Mum drinks a lot, stumbles upstairs where I'm probably on the computer and starts yelling at Dad in his office next to my room for some unknown reason, that's when I'll get worried. People with Huntington's don't have a fully functioning 'stop' button in their heads, so will just keep drinking until the bottle or bottles have all gone. And if they get angry at someone, which they can do very suddenly and with no warning, they just rage and rage at them. It's relentless. They also tend to take their frustration out on one particular person and go after that person when they are angry. For Mum it's usually Dad. Luckily Dad has ways of steering away any fights and avoiding letting things get out of hand. But everyone has a limit and there have been occasions where I just prefer to lock myself away with some loud music to drown out what's going on.

Even then it's only the occasional night where things go wrong and tempers get frayed. After a good sleep, wake up in the morning – all right, afternoon if possible – and everything's back to normal. Why should I drag my feelings from last night into a bright and shiny day? I simply choose not to. Things that bother me are events and the bother I feel gets wrapped in those moments. And then you get rid of them. A useful mental image I use is throwing them out of the window into a volcano, where they explode into thousands of little pieces. I enjoy explosions.

The slow worsening of the illness allows me time to strengthen to deal with it. As it grows, so do I and I'm keeping up at a rate which prevents it from getting to me. I know if I need them, Dad, Brom or Chan will leap to the rescue. Which they do nearly every day as it is.

I have mentioned the occasional argument more than once now. I believe this would be a good time to chuck in a few tips that I've picked up.

Top tips: family arguments

As you'll have gathered, there's the (more than) occasional time in our household when tensions get too high and people begin shouting. This doesn't just happen in homes with HD, of course; lots of people have to deal with arguments inside their own home. This is my advice for when it happens:

1. Remain calm. When you hear an argument going on downstairs, the worst thing you can do is run downstairs screaming your head off telling people to shut up because it's your home, too, and you have a right to live in peace. Adding to shouting solves nothing. I know. I've tried it. It doesn't work.

    If Mum's angry and getting angrier, the best way around it is for either my dad, or in some cases myself, to calm her without resorting to fighting back or contradicting her. Finding control inside yourself is challenging, but it's a useful talent that can stop heated debates and things escalating. People can get very fiery when they have Huntington's.

2. Ask for help. Don't be afraid to turn to a sibling, a grandparent, anyone who's capable of easing things. It should never be your burden alone. Countless times my brother and my grandma have found ways to settle arguments, and I rarely find myself at a point where there's no one to turn to.

3. Release your feelings. Crying is fine, laughing is good, and hitting things (like punchbags and pillows I mean, not breakable things or people's heads) depletes your anger. Keeping emotions pent up inside is dangerous and will lead to outbursts against people or things that do not deserve it. Let it out.

That's not a lot of tips to remember. In fact, you may find they're completely obvious. But this is how I cope when I hear my mum's voice rising, or when a door slams, etc.

Lack of memories

It's at times like that – the flare-ups I just referred to in the paragraphs above – when I realize just how far the Huntington's Disease has affected my mum's life and my own at the same time. I sometimes try to summon a mental image of my mother as she was before the illness set in. There's nothing.

I feel sick even now as I'm typing this very thought, but it's true. A few years ago, one of those rare occasions when my brother and I were left alone in the house for New Year, I told him that I was having difficulties bringing back memories of Mum being still when she wanted to be, of being able to walk around without stumbling. With all the comforting lines that he normally provides me with, it was odd to hear him say this one, and it has stayed in the back of my mind for years now. 'It sucks for you, dude, you've never known her.'

Of course he was a little drunk (it was New Year's Eve, remember), but it was something that was clearly lodged in both our heads. Could it be that I have never known my mother without the personality changing effects of HD? Have I not seen her walk a straight line before? Of course I have and I know it. It's just that my memory fails to serve me well by filling in all of those times with her as I see her now. In our memory we often see people as they are now rather than as they were.

My mother was…my mother *is* a caring, loving, incredible parent and always will be, no matter what. I've always been with the real her. I just sometimes forget it. She still has her great sense of humour, her love and her hope.

Mind the GAP

Here's an example of my mum's sense of humour.

'You sure this is all right, Danny?' Chris asked as he kicked his trainers off onto the small mat lying next to our front door. 'We're always invading your house.' I laughed with him and followed him into the living room. 'Of course it is! My parents are cool about a house full of teenagers. Not like we're throwing a party or anything is it?'

Chris slumped down onto the large sofa, cuddling up as usual to his girlfriend, whilst Abbi and Becca filled up the rest of the room by lounging across the other sofas in a typical teenage sprawl. I passed around the snacks, and whilst I was thinking of what DVD we should put on, Mum walked into the room. Abbi and Becca lit up instantly; both of them love talking to her about stuff, including jewellery, Johnny Depp, clothes, Johnny Depp, make-up and more Johnny Depp. She perched on the free spot next to me across from them and instantly a discussion of their favourite celebrity sparked off.

'I got no presents from Phil for Christmas,' Mum laughed, as I rolled my eyes at the coming joke. 'All my stuff was from Johnny Depp!' It was true. Dad had signed every gift he gave her from the man himself, as she absolutely loves Johnny Depp. Needless to say half of what she got had his face sprawled across it in one place or another – calendars, posters, books, all with Johnny Depp on the front. As expected, Abbi and Becca burst into fits of laughter and began discussing his 'dreaminess', in which Chris, his girlfriend and I lost all interest. I laughed with my mum though; it was really lovely to see her so happy and energetic, which she always is in company. It's being stuck on her own she hates.

'Do you two know about this GAP thing then?' she blurted out. I froze. During the Christmas celebrations I had somehow told her about GAP (the clothes label) supposedly standing for 'Gay and Proud', either in teenage mythology or for real, I don't know which. The fact I was wearing a t-shirt with the letters imprinted boldly on one sleeve did not help as I knew what was coming.

'GAP thing?' Abbi asked.

'The "Gay pride"!' Mum chuckled. 'Danny told me about it standing for...'

'Gay and Proud,' I muttered, rolling my eyes.

'That's it,' she shouted. The girls seemed to be enjoying seeing my face burning. It was at this point she decided to turn to me and say: 'Danny, I don't mind if you come home gay, so long as you don't come home pregnant!'

Even I could not restrain a smile as everybody in the room fell about laughing, lasting for a good half a minute before finally calming down to the occasional giggle in the background. 'So, who wants to watch a movie?' I said quickly, before I could be the butt of yet more mum jokes. I jammed *Edward Scissorhands* into the DVD player and switched it on as quickly as possible.

So, yes, I do know the real her: I see it in moments like that. She loves company, especially young people, joking and enjoying life. She's laid-back yet challenging and has a mischievous sense of humour.

Set yourself free

While I am happy for Brom and Chan (his wife), who left recently for a new life in London, it's hard not to feel slightly jealous at the same time, which I hate myself for. Living over an hour away certainly makes the distance feel huge, distancing yourself from these particular troubles in life, though that wasn't the intention of course.

I know it's harsh of me, because they must feel guilty too for leaving the three of us behind. We all see each other at least once a month, if not more, but it never does feel like enough and I'm often annoyed that we only spend a few hours together before vanishing back home. At the same time I need to leave them to their new lives, which is what I really want for them deep down. I may still be in this house and experiencing HD firsthand every day, but I have my own coping mechanisms; places to retreat in my head where there isn't any evidence of HD around.

I love to write, for example. I haven't stopped writing since I was about eight. I remember the first long story I wrote was back in Year 4 when I was just eight years old. My fantastic teacher was handing around photographs, with the one simple task: write a story to do with this picture. Mine was a harbour, with boats bobbing up and down gently on the sea. At the time I was completely stumped, since I had never tried writing stories properly before then and I had no clue what was expected of me. So I started writing.

A few months later I was reading out page 40 to the class, delighted at my friends' reactions, for I had chosen them all as characters. Instead of focusing on the harbour, I'd written about one of the boats, about a sailing trip ending in a disastrous crash on a remote island. There were about ten characters, far too many for a book, all of them having many comical adventures.

Since then I've never been without some kind of writing project. It's moved from 'Shipwreck' – my first long story – to a competition story about a little girl and a dragon (that story gave me one of my best days ever, because I won a national competition with it), a complex War Hammer-type story about Dark Elves and, most recently, a sci-fi book with characters once again based on my friends.

I find it so easy to get lost in these worlds, to become absorbed in the characters and drift off with them, watching events through their eyes and helping them grow. Writing is one of my forms of freedom, a way of losing myself and withdrawing from the constant noise of the outer world, because it's a new land, a new universe which I control.

If you're not into the literary word, try music instead. According to my friends I have the strangest taste in music, since I find myself listening to classical, indie rock, sometimes orchestral tracks, maybe even the occasional heavy rock track, depending on my mood.

Once again it is easy to become lost in music, to let yourself be absorbed by the melodies and flow of the song. It's also why I find such joy in the piano. As I heard someone else say who plays piano, no other instrument has ever made me feel so connected with my emotions. I've tried the clarinet and the guitar, but the piano lets you express yourself. This getting too soppy? Tough. Sometimes emotions do tend to creep up on people and it's important to have some outlet. Letting your happiness, depression or rage leak out in creativity is that outlet for me. I'd draw if I could…but my prowess with a pencil only goes as far as stick figures.

Telling others

Another issue that comes up a lot nowadays for me is deciding how I am going to tell my friends about HD. It's not a very easy decision, since most of the time I'd rather they not know at all; I despise being pitied. However, when they're coming around my house or are asking why it is I'm in such a mood, sometimes there's no way around the answer and I just have to be honest. I've had some varying reactions over the years as I've let people know my secret.

Some just nod. I'm not sure if this is because they don't quite get it, or if they're just the kind of person who can take things in their stride. Either way these people tend to be the easiest to get along with, even if there is a nagging sensation in the back of your mind that they haven't actually 'got' what you just said.

Others start with 'Oh, I'm so sorry,' and eventually stop after five minutes of you asking them to be quiet. It's very kind that people care so much but to be honest I've heard it all before. I'm not telling them for the sympathy so most of the time it's quite annoying, if anything.

Once I had a girl burst into tears. Since it was over the online chatting system MSN Messenger, this was highly odd, meaning I really had absolutely nothing to do but wait for it all to subside. I've never had someone cry virtual tears online before or since. Luckily no one's got that upset in person, because I'd have absolutely no clue how I would calm them down. A pat on the back, maybe. Maybe my timing was just terrible with that one. It's all a matter of timing and your own judgement about whether or not the person is ready to learn about what is hanging over your life.

The main thing people tend to get wrong is that 'this disease has taken over my life'. Check your facts. It's only a part of my life! A lot of times I've felt like maybe I shouldn't be with the great friends I have today because of what may happen to me in the future, that I wouldn't want to drag them down by feeling miserable if the worst happens. But I've still managed to hang on to them regardless.

Summer camps

A few years ago I was escorted to the Huntington's Summer Camp. I say escorted, what I mean was dragged out of the house kicking and screaming; I'm very much a hermit crab, and a weekend with a total bunch of strangers was not about to be my top priority for summer. I'm still not 100 per cent sure why I was even made to go there in the first place, but sure enough as soon as school broke up I was driven down to the New Forest and taken into a huge manor, of sorts. After fiddling around with papers and finding the entrance, I said goodbye to my parents and was taken into my dorm where I met a group of other boys.

Most of them were older than me, a couple of the same age and only two any younger. For the first few hours I felt completely out of my element; the lot of us were being thrown all over the premises for various activities, and I had only just unpacked. Everyone got on with one another and seemed to know each other, which meant I was spending most of my time standing around gawking.

But it did not last long. The activities were amazingly fun, including venturing around trees with just a rope strapped to your waist as a life-line, swimming in the outdoor pool and archery. Only two short days but they were full of fun. I definitely made some decent friends whilst I was there, though I only returned once more and afterwards never went back. What was funny was it was a trip for people with Huntington's in the family, but it made you completely forget about it in the process.

A life of clutter

The symptoms of Mum's disease often make things messy around the home. But, since I'm a teenager with a typical teenage room (the kind of person who can't find the floor in his own bedroom because of the mess), it doesn't bother me. Mum drops things a lot, so there's often a mess on the floor, normally yoghurt or occasionally a broken glass. The washing up seems to have tripled in the past year, and there's an eternal mess around where she likes to sit and smoke, at the end of the dining table.

Smoking is constant and often a window or the front door has to be left open so that the room gets aired out. We've had to buy an ashtray with a small fan inserted inside, which still manages to get clogged and die every other week, and buy a large 'air-swapping machine', the only way I can describe it. It seems to purify the air, since about half a year ago it was nearly impossible for me to sit downstairs and watch TV since you could just *see* the layers of smoke drifting across the room.

Luckily we're adapting. I'm still a nightmare when it comes to cleaning, as Brom, Chan and Dad will no doubt mention, since I rarely offer a helping hand. Sometimes I look away if Mum knocks her drink onto the floor accidentally, because if I bend down to pick it up it makes me look like I'm picking up after her – which I would be – and I know she hates people fussing around her. I'd hate to make her think that I'm going to end up becoming a carer for her too, so I try not to do anything until she's left the room or if the thing she's dropped is dangerous, like a burning cigarette. That's my excuse, anyway, for not joining in with the constant cleaning and picking up of spilt things. Dad says the excuse is wearing a bit thin.

Mum has got quieter over the years and finds it harder to join in conversations. She gets very tired sometimes and will sit in silence or get lost in a book and not notice you come in – people with Huntington's can focus very hard on one thing to the exclusion of all else. So, I have to start the conversations when I walk in from school. Years ago she'd yell, 'Hi Danny, how are you?' as soon as the front door clicked shut, but now the Huntington's gets in the way so the loud greeting comes from me.

When she's particularly tired there's also a difficulty in her speech, as words become slurred and she sometimes has to stop mid-sentence to think about what she is going to say next. I get annoyed at other people when they don't give her a chance to finish her sentence. You have to slow the conversation down to her pace and give her space to say what she wants to.

Once or twice, when she's trying to speak across the table when guests are over and she's had to struggle with a sentence a few times, I say it for her absent-mindedly. I don't mean to be rude, since I hate to interrupt her. I especially don't want her feeling that she can't do simple things like that for herself either, but at the same time it's nice to know I have that connection with her still. The HD hasn't taken that away from us.

Also, Mum can't drive any more. It was disastrous to come home from school and see her in tears, having just lost her licence. I had no words; I just gave her a huge hug and told her everything would be all right. Now Dad has to take her shopping, to the local newsagents for cigarettes and other supplies. So, she has substituted Charlie the horse for the little sporty car she used to love driving, and rides him across fields instead, with Jo or Dad running alongside, trying to keep up in case she falls off. Mum doesn't give up on her freedom and independence; she just finds other ways of expressing it if her usual way gets taken away from her.

Other people

My awareness of how other people see us has been on a steady rise as Mum's condition decreases. The most annoying times, for me, are when we have to go to a supermarket or a restaurant. Wandering around the aisles is the kind of nightmare that I want to end fast. I'm so thankful that Mum is so strong, as she continues to hurl herself down the shop and grab the items we need with confidence and strength.

Meanwhile, I trail along behind her, hating the whole shopping thing for two reasons: (1) I'm a teenager and (2) other people staring! To be fair, most people don't stare. But rude ones do. I cannot stand staring. I wish they would all just have some sense and get on with their own business. I am always impressed with the way Mum ignores people's stares and does not let them limit what she wants to do.

Dad and my grandma Maggie are now responsible for taking her to the shops since she cannot go by herself any more, meaning I have to go less and less now. Still, the occasional trips leave me fuming. I find great pleasure in glaring dirtily at anyone who has refused to tear their eyes away. I seem to have perfected it, since the last man staggered backwards, grabbed his bread and strode off without a second glance.

End, or rather beginning

There's a lot going on in my life at the moment – exams at school, acting in a play, writing stories, doing things with my friends – but this seems almost minor, in terms of impact on my life, compared with what I've got coming in a few years. That's what you have to avoid: allowing your possible future to overshadow your actual present and stop you enjoying it.

The genetic test I plan to take at 18 is the only test I ever hope to fail. Also sitting there in the future waiting for us is the prospect that HD is just going to continue to worsen for Mum. That all may seem pretty bleak. However, scientists across the globe are throwing research into finding treatments and a cure for Huntington's, and they seem to be getting close on a number of fronts. Both my parents are confident that it doesn't matter if either Brom or I get the disease anyway, as at the rate things are going at the moment there'll be a cure in no time. Though that's what they've been saying for years since scientists discovered the faulty gene.

A clearer hope for the future is present within the close, supportive family I've got, rather than in the chance of a cure being developed. Of course when you are tired or down, you always have worries nagging away at the back of your mind. One of them is what's going to happen between my parents. They do care for each other. Yet there may come a stage where there might honestly not be a lot left in the two of them. These past few years have been incredibly hard on both my mum and dad, since they've had to learn to accept the harsh truth, cope with a new life and alter everything. Both seem emotionally, physically and mentally drained at times.

There's always a chance that the two of them will not be able to stay together any more, possibly after I have gone off to college or left home afterwards to find my own flat and live my own life. However, though things sometimes look bad, like when there is bad news about a drug trial that didn't have the positive effect on Mum's symptoms that we all hoped, for example, things can always get better. Just because the sun has set does not mean it's never going to rise again. We all try to learn to accept life as it comes, grow even stronger and continue to live as we do now, still laughing at the simple things and loving those near to us.

Living. It's as simple as breathing, yet it can be the hardest task of all. Hope is what keeps me going, a hope that there will be a cure, that my family is going to live on as close as we are now, enjoying every moment we can spend together: hope restored by my friends when all seems lost; hope reborn with songs and stories; hope that will never die even if the shadow over our future continues to darken. Because there's not a chance in hell that I'm going to let it.

CHAPTER 5

Eyes Wide Open: The Daughter-in-law's Story

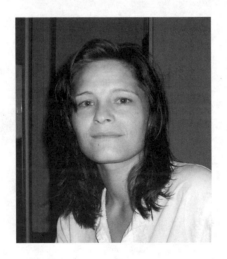

G'day. My name's Chantel and I'm 28 years old. I've been married to Bromley, Sandy's older son, for two years and we live in London. It's a far cry from where I grew up, a suburb of Melbourne, Australia, but I enjoy it mostly. I'm not a big fan of the Tube to be honest, especially in summer. I miss the beaches back home too. And Dad's infamous BBQs and my favourite brand of lager and…enough of that. I'll make myself homesick. Really, I do like living here and I'm lucky that I have a job that I love too. I'm a children's bookseller and I get to read kids' books all the time, which is great. They have a simple honesty and innocence that adult books don't.

So, why is this so hard to write?

To be honest I'm finding it hard to write this because half the members of the family are journalists or natural born writers. With all the books I read I was hoping some of it would rub off on me but unfortunately I'm as inarticulate as ever. So if you're willing to put up with me I'll try to tell you my part in this family story.

When Sandy and Phil pitched this book idea to the family I thought, 'Great. No one's really written much about the effects of Huntington's on an entire family before and it might be good therapy for everyone to get stuff off their chests.' I jumped in whole-heartedly. In reality I've found it bloody hard to write anything.

If we'd written this two years ago when Brom and I lived in their house I'd have found it easy, surrounded by the constant mess and tidying, the drinking and the mood swings that take place, seemingly, in the blink of an eye. Then there was also the frustration and anger (on my part) caused by the littlest things. It used to drive me crazy. And the worst part was it wasn't anyone's fault. There was no one to blame. HD caused those unpleasant feelings and for a while controlled our daily lives.

Now that we live away from the family home I find it hard to recall those feelings. I think that's a good thing. I didn't like feeling so angry and upset all the time over something I couldn't really control. Living in a house with Huntington's Disease also used to make me constantly think whether this would be our possible future, I mean Brom and me, and naturally that was upsetting.

Where I come from

I come from a dysfunctional but relatively 'normal' family. My parents split up when I was 11 or 12 and my two brothers were nine and six. It hurt for a while but life went on. My dad did a brilliant job bringing up my two brothers and me on his own. He provided everything he could and I've never felt we missed out on anything, not important things anyway. (There is still the matter of a family holiday to Queensland he promised us 10 years ago!)

Anyway eventually both my parents met other people and we became one big happy extended family. As a kid I'd always wanted a sister. When Dad remarried I got four. I also gained another two brothers from Mum's second marriage. Just call us the Brady Bunch.

Five and a half years ago I came to the UK with friends to do some travelling, see the sights and have some fun. One week after landing I was in the town of Banbury, 20 miles north-west of Oxford, working in a bar. A couple of weeks later I met Brom and we got talking over a few drinks. We still argue over who hit on who but I know with perfect clarity the moment I fell in love with him. It was one of the happiest yet scariest moments of my life. One thing led to another and here we are five years later married, much to my mother's shame. Before I came over here she had said the worst thing I could do in life was to fall in love with an Englishman I'd met in a pub. (She adores him now though!)

I don't remember where we were the first time Brom mentioned that his mum had Huntington's Disease (in a pub again no doubt) but I remember the look on his face when I said I knew what it was before he'd had a chance to explain it. He looked kinda relieved that he didn't have to explain it to me and at the same time a little apprehensive as to what I might say next or what questions I might ask. I could see that the whole topic had made him feel uncomfortable. To be honest I felt a little queasy too.

In my last year of school I studied biology and our major assignment was to do a comprehensive study of a genetic disorder. I chose to study Huntington's Disease. We had to explain what the disease was, how it affected sufferers, and what treatment was available to help combat the disease. As I began researching I started getting quite depressed reading about the mental and physical effects on a sufferer and the fact that it was totally incurable. I felt sick to my stomach reading case studies. What a horrible thing to have to go through. So, having studied all that, when Brom told me about his mum, I didn't ask any questions and we changed the subject.

Meeting the scary in-laws

The first time I met Sandy and Phil I was pretty scared. This was mostly due to all the usual reasons people worry before meeting their partner's parents. Would they like me and would we get along OK? Brom had told me that Sandy often didn't like his girlfriends and I knew that he and Phil were going through a rough period. I was also a little worried about how I would react to Huntington's. Even though I had studied the disease at school I hadn't met someone with it.

We hadn't really talked much more about it so I was unsure what to expect. Brom had explained that the disease was still showing in its early stages. He warned me about the sudden movements that Sandy sometimes made and to maybe stand a little way off. I later learnt this lesson the hard way through intensive headaches from being head-butted by accident. I wish now I had shares in an ibuprofen company. He also mentioned that she sometimes forgot little things. Before meeting Sandy I never drank tea. I would always ask for coffee if she offered. But she'd forget and make me a tea instead. It took me a while to get used to, but I love a good cup of tea now.

Sandy and I got on really well. It's hard not to like her. She has a wicked sense of humour and she's very open and easy-going. Sandy, Phil and Danny treated me like a member of the family and I'm really thankful for that because I was so far away from home and missed my own family quite a bit in those early days.

For a year or so Brom and I moved around travelling and working and we had lots of fun. I think for Brom it was a nice escape from the increasingly turbulent home life and a chance to get out and find who he really was inside, away from Huntington's. He matured a lot during that period and seemed to become a lot more comfortable within himself.

Living with HD: the test run

Pretty soon my two years in the UK were up. A few months before my visa expired and I had to return to Australia, Brom decided he'd come along too. Phil and Sandy offered for us both to live with them so we could save some money for the trip and spend some time with them before disappearing for a year.

I've come to realize that moving in with the family was as beneficial to them as it was to us. We helped redecorate quite a bit of the house. A fresh coat of paint on the walls and lots of de-cluttering are what I remember most from that period. Oh, and the constant, never-ending cleaning and tidying of course. If Extreme Cleaning ever becomes one of those strange extreme sports (apparently, Extreme Ironing is now a sport), we'll win as we've become experts. Cleaning has got to be *the* worst superficial side effect of HD.

I also spent a lot of time with Sandy, shopping mostly. This I enjoyed, except when people would stare and sometimes point as she walked past. I don't know if Sandy notices but I do and it used to make my blood boil. I would glare at people, willing them to make a snide remark, just so I could yell at them and tell them how rude and ignorant they were being. It was quite pointless really, though. If Sandy does notice then she doesn't show that she cares, so why should I, and I know she wouldn't want me to be upset about it.

Living with the family during that period was highly stressful at times. I got frustrated at everything and anything. I often got quite angry at nothing in particular and found myself taking it out on Brom, which was unfair. Sometimes there were arguments, which, again, were pointless. Who's to blame? No one.

It wasn't always doom and gloom though. I'm just pointing out a few bad bits. The majority of the time it was a fun place to be, with lots of laughs and quality family time together. I particularly remember Saturday nights when Phil would cook dinner. Some old 1980s record would be playing and the rest of us would be sitting around the lounge room chilling out, reading and playing computer games. When dinner was ready we'd all sit down together to eat.

Looking back now I think of that period as a kind of test. Until this time I hadn't really thought seriously about Huntington's or how it might affect my life. Brom and I knew we wanted to be together and I knew there was a 50 per cent chance he could inherit the disease but I hadn't really considered what that meant for our future.

Back to the other side of the world

When we left to spend a year back in Australia with my family it was kind of a relief to some extent, a chance to relax and not live with HD staring us in the face 24/7. I think we pretty much forgot all about it. But the year went quickly and it was too soon when Brom had to come back to the UK. By now we knew our future together lay in England due to Sandy having HD. There was no way I could ask Brom to stay on in Australia so I stayed behind and applied for a common-law partner visa because we'd been together three years at this point. It was rejected on the grounds of lack of evidence.

I'll never forget the phone call to Brom to tell him the bad news. It was horrible, except it was also brilliant. We decided to get married, a bit earlier than planned but we knew it would work out.

My family were really happy for us. They all love Brom to bits and were really happy that he was joining our family. They'd also met Sandy, Phil and Danny earlier that year when they came over to Australia for a holiday. Brom and I had mentioned the HD and what to expect but they didn't bat an eyelid. I wasn't surprised that our families got along so well for those two weeks. It was great that our folks got to meet at least once considering the distances involved.

One thing that did surprise me though was my youngest brother's reaction one night when we were all out together at the Casino in Melbourne. Someone had pointed to Sandy and made a snide comment about her being 'wasted' because of the way she stumbles sometimes when walking. Stephen (my brother) got very angry and shot off a few swear words at the ignorant bastard, who looked suitably shocked and just a little ashamed. For the rest of the night Stephen took it upon himself to be a kind of bodyguard to Sandy. He was constantly on the lookout, and ready to step in if anyone so much as glanced in her direction.

He was only doing what we've all done in the past but I was surprised by how much it seemed to affect him emotionally considering he'd only met Sandy the week before. I'm guessing it was partly due to how much he liked Brom and he felt he was protecting Sandy on his behalf. Because of this incident I've always felt that amongst my family Stephen has the strongest understanding of how HD affects us all here. I'm not sure they fully comprehend what's involved, but then who does if they're not in direct contact with it on a daily basis? This isn't to say that when the chips are down and *if* Brom is unlucky enough to develop HD they won't be there for us. I know they will.

It's a shame we don't all live in one place. I'm sure we'd hang out together a lot and I think my folks would be a good source of support and friendship for Sandy and Phil.

What Brom said before we were married

Brom has only once tried to give me a chance to walk away from HD and the possible future it may bestow upon us. One night the week before the wedding he sat me down and asked if I was really sure I wanted to marry him. If he has inherited the disease our future will be full of hardships and added stress that he feels I shouldn't have to live with.

Naturally I said yes, I was sure. I didn't feel there was a choice to make. I love him and that is more important than any stupid disease and the havoc it may cause one day in the future. How selfish would I be to turn my back on him when he will need me the most? He accepted my answer but did say that if he finds he does have the disease he will leave me. This hurt a lot. I understand his reasoning though. He's worried that he'll become violent towards me or that I'll resent him and our relationship if I end up becoming his primary carer one day. I think maybe that he'd also feel ashamed that he couldn't look after me the way he wants to. He's very protective and sometimes old-fashioned in that way.

To test or not to test

Some days I think our lives would be easier if Brom had the test to see if he has the HD gene. If it came back positive we could organize our future plans a little, factor the illness into the dreams of having a family, a nice house and a secure lifestyle. When we hopefully have kids one day we could have the embryo tested to ensure the child wouldn't have the disease too. Or we could try IVF. They can implant HD-free swimmers and we could breed it out of the family line so to speak.

And, yet, if the test came back positive it would probably ruin Brom's life and state of mind. It would be a massive blow to his confidence and self-esteem. It would be like a prolonged death sentence. Imagine trying to live your life, succeed and enjoy yourself while at the same time just waiting for the symptoms to manifest themselves. He'd probably have a nervous breakdown. I think I would too.

On the other hand there's also the prospect of a test coming back negative. The relief would be immense. We could live a normal life, have kids and happily drive each other nuts for the rest of our lives. But (there's always a but with HD) that would leave Brom's brother Danny on his own in being at risk. I know that the possibility of his younger brother getting the illness is something that scares Brom even more than if he himself had HD. I think he'd feel guilty (that protective thing again). This probably sounds a bit odd but, if one of them ends up with it, in a way we both hope Brom is the one and Danny gets the all clear. We have a strong relationship-marriage-friendship and we know we'd get through it together. Not to say that Danny won't have this with a partner one day too. We just don't want to watch HD happen to him.

So what I'm trying to say is that I totally respect Brom's decision not to have the test. The possible outcomes are just too stressful and we don't need that.

A luckier generation

We are lucky, in a way, compared with Sandy and Phil and with Sandy's parents before her. Fifteen years ago people with HD were quite often misdiagnosed (as Sandy's dad was) and as a consequence, sufferers were possibly not given the best medicines or treatment to help combat the symptoms. But in the mid-1990s the gene that causes HD was discovered and there has been a flurry of research into treatments and possible cures since then. Today HD is a widely recognized disease the world over and amazing research is being conducted into how to deal with the symptoms. By the time either Brom or Danny might develop the symptoms there could even be a cure.

At the very least we've had the opportunity to watch how the disease develops and are hopefully better equipped to deal with it in our own futures. It's as if Sandy's generation of sufferers are the guinea pigs, going through constant tests, drug trials and more tests, finding the right diet, the right exercise regimes for the muscles, the right emotional and mental state to help them cope. We can look at what works and what doesn't and hopefully use it to our advantage if necessary.

Having been part of this family for a while now, I've watched them all change in ways they might not have noticed themselves. Apart from Sandy that is. The physical changes are quite obvious as the disease continues to develop but mentally she is the only one who's remained the same in some respects. Five years ago she was a happy, chirpy person who was game for anything and always up for a laugh and she is still that way today.

Individually, each member seems more confident and more relaxed. As a unit the family is stronger, happier and better able to deal with HD. I guess this has something to do with learning how to roll with the punches and take each day as a blessing of sorts.

Brom and I have a much more relaxed lifestyle now, living away from the family home. Brom's studying, I'm working in a job I enjoy and we get lots of time to spend together. We often feel guilty that we don't help out as much as we used to or probably should but we can't put our lives on hold. We've got plans. When Brom's finished university and gained the work experience he wants, we're going to move back to Australia and set up home and business, have a family, travel and do whatever else takes our fancy. These things may or may not happen but if we didn't have these hopes and dreams we'd get pretty miserable.

We've all got our own methods of coping and stopping ourselves from sinking into depression or the 'poor me, poor us, it's not fair' syndrome. If I feel a bit down I remind myself that there is always someone worse off than myself, like starving children in Africa who have been orphaned by AIDS or millions of people across the world with no access to fresh, clean water, no roof over their heads and nothing on their dinner plates. These aren't the most pleasant thoughts to have but they always make me realize how lucky I am.

You can't live a life of 'what ifs'

And every day I think about how lucky I am to have Brom. He's the kindest, funniest person I know and he's my best friend. He may inherit HD one day and I can't deny that the thought scares the hell out of me. I'm not ready to lose him now and I won't be ready or willing then either. But I know it will be OK whatever happens. We've got each other, our families and a handful of the best friends you could ever want.

And I think we've got the right attitudes too. We know that you can't live a life of 'what ifs'. If it does happen, we'll fight it. We'll make our life as comfortable as possible and we'll remember to always try to see the funny side of life. Either way, we'll deal with what happens. We'll strive to enjoy every moment we can together, be it 25 years with HD or 60-odd years without.

CHAPTER 6

Mopping the Ceiling: The Husband's Story

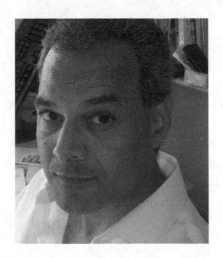

I'm Phil, Sandy's husband. I'm 46. We've been together almost 24 years, apart from a six-month gap ten years ago. We have two sons. Bromley, 25, is my step-son (Sandy was married before). But I've been his acting dad since his age was measured in months rather than years. Danny is 15. Bromley was married two years ago to the newest member of our family, Chantel, who is from Australia and has made his life very happy. Bromley and Chantel now live in London. Danny, Sandy and I live in a village in Oxfordshire, about 85 miles outside London. Sandy has Huntington's Disease. The boys are each 50 per cent at risk of inheriting it.

So, that's the scene-setting done. This chapter is written in bits, because there's never time to do anything properly with Huntington's Disease in the family. Just to prove it, I can hear a glass smashing downstairs, so I'll be back in a minute. While I'm clearing up whatever smashed, I'll leave you to read this email exchange I just had with a friend whose partner also has Huntington's Disease. The symptoms have only recently started to become significant with them, so they are a few years behind us.

In a message dated 01/08/2006 00:54:56:

Mariah to Phil

Hey,

Just finished reading your draft chapter. Thanks for sharing it.
   I feel so small and Huntington's is so massive I feel awestruck by it, paralysed. I want to do the best I can for Steve, but I don't know where I will find the strength to deal with it when it gets to the stage you are at with Sandy. I'm terrified.

Mariah

In a message dated 02/08/2006 02:25:20:

Phil to Mariah

Hi

Don't be awe-struck. I didn't/don't think I had it in me either – don't on bad days and didn't until recently.
   Up until about a year or two ago I was terrified by this whole thing. I spent most of my time pretending to

cope so I didn't frighten the boys too much. I was waiting for the one incident that would be the straw that broke the camel's back, where I would just cave in and not be any use to anyone any more.

I don't know exactly what happened – got sick of being scared I think. But some kind of calm settled on me a year or two ago. I stopped looking around in a panic thinking, 'Where's the responsible adult who can really deal with this, since I'm just pretending?' and accepted that there's just me and I'll have to do.

It's not always there – on bad days calm is the last thing I am. But my steady state has gone (mostly) from panic to calm. And that means it's easier to cope with 'incidents' as Dan calls them, when things get fraught, because there's some respite in between where you can gather your energies back.

I think it is at least partly because Dan is so upbeat and doing well and Brom has pulled himself back from the crappy years he had in his late teens. He and Chantel are happy, he is doing well at college – all the things he used to think weren't for him are going right. Seeing the boys turn out so strong and capable and knowing they are enjoying life has helped me move away from being on the edge of panic.

So, maybe I'm just reacting to circumstance, I don't know. But, if I can do it, anyone can do it.

Things can get better. You can get past the panic. Honest. Hang in there,

Phil

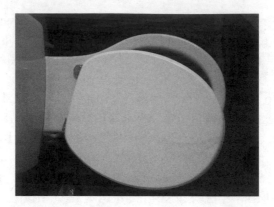

Things fall apart

Back again. All cleared up and no harm done. Interesting new yogurt stain on the living room carpet, though. It'll blend in with the other stains over time. And the zig-zag pattern of the cigarette burns in the carpet offset it quite nicely. I just passed the bathroom on the way back to the office, where I am writing this, and thought you should see what I just saw.

I hadn't intended to start this chapter with a toilet seat, but when you are living with Huntington's Disease in the family you soon learn that things never go as intended. So I'll have to appeal to you to just go with the flow. I have to, and it will show through in the disjointed nature of this chapter. Art imitating life and all that. Or is that supposed to be the other way round? Let's blame that confusion on the permanently frazzled state your mind settles into when you are living with HD in the house. Huntington's needs constant low-level maintenance. It's forever tapping you on the shoulder or tugging on your shirt sleeve, leaving you with what sometimes feels like attention-deficit disorder.

So, back to the loo seat. I expect your toilet seat lid doesn't have such a rakish angle to it. It's probably perched primly and properly above the seat, like all well-behaved toilet seat lids should be, rather than looking as if it's trying to free itself and escape out the door, as ours does.

This is our fifth toilet seat in seven months. There is, as you'll have worked out from that fact, no great life expectancy to toilet seats in our house. They are doomed to a short and brutal existence as soon as they are carried in through the front door. I'm thinking of starting to buy them in bulk, maybe wholesale or something. One of the metal hinges on this latest one snapped due to the force with which the lid was repeatedly slammed down. Hence its crazy angle.

The fabric of our house is possibly the most unexpected casualty of HD and the one people talk about least. I am about to go on about it for a few paragraphs, partly because we spend a lot of time inside this house, so it's part of the daily landscape, partly because it's been our family home for 13 years and so is the backdrop to much of our life and the stage on which our dramas are played out, and partly, I suspect, because it's easier to write about the impact of Huntington's Disease on our home than about its impact on ourselves.

Unexpected early casualties

Huntington's shapes your environment in surprising ways. In fact, the house began to bear scars inflicted by Huntington's Disease before we even knew we were living with HD. It's as if our home was acting out something for us, reflecting with surface wear and tear some of the emotional damage we were all (the family members, that is) going through on the inside. I know that's fanciful, but I don't get out much. The impact of HD on the house used to puzzle me, appearing like crop circles overnight, to be discovered in the morning when you are most bleary-eyed, in need of coffee, and your brain is particularly slow at processing the unexpected.

There is a clock on the wall in our kitchen, for example. It's a cheap, yellow, plastic-framed clock. I looked up at it as I was filling the kettle the other day and noticed that the left half of the plastic surround was riddled with holes. I stared at it, confused, as the kettle started to overflow into the sink. Plastic-eating mice? Plastic-eating mice that can scale walls? My brain gave up.

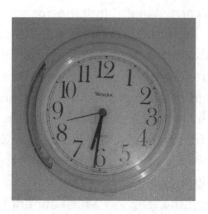

Once there were handles

I'll give you a further tour of the kitchen so you can get a sense of how HD chips away at its surroundings. We have a glass oven door. On several occasions the door spontaneously and mysteriously came away off its weakened hinges and crashed to the floor, once shattering into a thousand pieces. I found what was left of the door in the morning, just before I stepped on it. As an aside, but continuing the theme of how slightly off-beam life is with HD in the family, that evening I found Sandy trying to cook a chicken in the oven, with no oven door. The heat hit you as soon as you walked into the kitchen. We had fish fingers instead.

I'd like you to notice the cupboards now, if you will. We have 12 kitchen cupboards. Each used to have a little knob or handle attached. Currently only six have a knob or handle. And they are of varying shapes and sizes. There is an ongoing sourcing and replacement programme for the knobs carried out, obviously not very efficiently, by me. One cupboard lacks its door and just gapes, showing off its tins of baked beans and packets of instant noodles to anyone who cares to glance that way and wonder where the door has gone.

It's in the garage, waiting to be re-hung. It's been waiting a year so far. Don't hold your breath. Then, over in the corner is the sleek-looking fridge-freezer, with no visible handles on the doors. Look closer. The absence of handles isn't actually a design feature. They were there when we bought it. But they snapped off years ago. We open the fridge, the freezer and the handle-less cupboards by scrabbling to get a hold on the edge of the respective door and then tugging.

Life is maintenance

The mysteries – what happened to the clock, why the oven door kept disintegrating, why the knobs and handles all break off – are eventually solved if you wait around and observe long enough. Sandy keeps her cigarettes in an overhead cupboard in the kitchen. A few days after noticing the shattered clock surround, I spotted Sandy walk into the room and fling the cupboard door open so she could retrieve a pack of cigarettes. That particular cupboard is one of the few still to have a knob on the door, a knob that crashed hard into the plastic clock on the wall, knocking yet another shard of plastic off it before the door swung back closed with a clunk. Mystery solved. Likewise the oven. Sandy stopped cooking a year or two ago. The oft-replaced oven door stopped coming apart in my hands about the same time.

We don't realize how much finesse we apply to the control of our muscles, the fine motor skills involved in closing a toilet seat without a loud crash or shutting an oven door without slamming it. It's a problem of amplitude. Someone with HD will hurl a glass oven door shut with the same amount of force they would apply to a heavy car door. The dial that controls muscle movements seems permanently set on full.

Brom, our older son, says his mum has super strength. I discovered more evidence of that this morning. The towel rail was on the floor of the cloakroom. It had been virtually welded onto the wall with as many different industrial strength adhesives as we could find, after it had hit the ground several times before. There was a liberal mix of No More Nails adhesive, super glue and that epoxy resin stuff that you mix together and then can suspend yourself from the ceiling with if you feel so inclined, all mixed together to keep the towel rail where it was supposed to be. You could sit on it if you wanted to. Or park a small elephant on it. Yet there it was, on the floor, with a towel rail shaped chunk of plaster gone from the wall, too. I think Brom has a point. No wonder we often tiptoe around Sandy to avoid getting her mad.

You can track where a person with HD is in a house by listening for the noises of household objects straining under pressure and sometimes giving way with a crack – the refrigerator door colliding at speed with the wall as it is flung open, or the occasional spectacular sound effect, such as the splintering of wood as a cupboard door is yanked off its hinges and crashes to the ground. You soon learn to ignore the day-to-day sounds and only get up to investigate when it's a particularly dramatic one. Or the sound of breaking glass. Or a smoke alarm. There is one in every room and a fire extinguisher on each floor. Danny even has an extinguisher in his room. Other kids have TVs. He has an extinguisher. Every few months I annoy him by reminding him how to use it.

The oddest sound that ever brought us running was an exploding glass ashtray. Apparently they can deal with the heat of one or two smouldering cigarettes. But, when there are ten or so burning merrily away in the bottom of the glass, as was the case on this occasion, they shatter. Brom and Chan were on the other side of the living room, watching a movie on TV. Brom's mum had gone to bed, leaving the little inferno building up to the heat of a thousand suns or whatever critical mass it takes to explode an ashtray. And then, at the climax of the film they were watching, it blew, leaving little flames licking away at the wooden table top. If they hadn't been there to put it out…well, I guess the smoke alarm would have told us and we would have got to use the extinguishers for real. As it was, Brom and Chan poured a glass of water on it.

'Life is maintenance,' I read somewhere recently. As I wander around with a screw driver at the end of each day, tightening the hinges on the cupboard doors – the perpetual banging loosens them and sends them crashing to the ground without regular preventive action – I have to agree.

Huntington's Disease impacts on your life and your surroundings in many small and varied ways. Taken individually, they are trivial. But if you let them, they can accumulate to clog up your life in a similar way to the accumulation of the tiny clumps of plaque that clog up the brain and cause the symptoms of Huntington's Disease in the first place. Which brings us to cleaning.

Mopping the ceiling

There's a character in the *Peanuts* cartoon strip who generates mess. One strip I remember shows him sitting still, doing nothing. In each panel, more and more mess has accumulated around him: things fall over, stains appear on his clothes, he becomes increasingly dishevelled. All without moving or doing anything. He appears oblivious to the mess and disorder accumulating around him. Flies start circulating above his head.

'We can't pay for house cleaning,' says the social worker, 'because cleaning isn't part of personal care.' We are sitting round our dining table, four of us. Carol, the HD Association's regional advisor, who has convened this meeting-at-home with our new social worker and is there to help fight our corner, glances at me, ready to jump in when needed. 'Whoever made up that rule hasn't lived with HD,' I say. 'There's a kind of tornado effect. Everything hits the ground: glasses, cups, tea, dinner, lamps, chairs.' In fact, the force exerted by a flung arm from someone with HD is so powerful, the ceiling often needs cleaning.

I used to think it was just the floor and the walls that were regularly pasted with food and drink, till I glanced up and saw strawberry milkshake all over the ceiling one day. It had formed a spectacular spray effect, as if Jackson Pollock had been in. I still haven't caught Sandy in the act of slamming her glass down on the table with the gravity-defying force that pastes half a glass of milkshake to the ceiling. So I'm not sure how it's done without breaking the laws of physics. But the results have appeared several times while I am out of the room.

Mopping the ceiling has a surreal feel to it, as if symbolic of the way Huntington's tends to turn your world upside down. The first time it happened, Danny and one of his friends walked in through the front door and into the front room. I was mopping the ceiling. The ceiling, not the floor. They looked at me and paused. I paused, mop-to-ceiling, staring back. 'Er, you won't tell your parents that Danny's dad mops the ceiling, will you, or they might not let you back,' I said. Like teenagers everywhere, faced with a parental attempt at humour, they ignored it and headed for the PlayStation.

'Actually,' said Carol to the social worker, back in the meeting, 'you can use a health argument for paying for the cleaning. You'd be surprised at how unhygienic, unsanitary even, it can get if the rate food is dropped isn't matched by the rate it's cleared up.' Hmmm, clever, I thought. The social worker raised an eyebrow and made a note.

Groundhog Day

Anyone who cleans knows that slight dip of the spirit you feel when you walk back into a room and find that the kitchen work surface or floor that you had left gleaming and spotless a few hours previously is now littered with used teabags, spilt and now congealed sugar and a patina of something sticky that you can't quite identify.

The difference with HD is just how accelerated this whole cycle becomes. Walk out of spotless kitchen and check answerphone messages in the home-office for ten minutes. Walk back in and your feet are sticking to something vaguely unpleasant on the floor; there's half a tin of sugar scattered across the work surface and, strangely, a knob of butter sitting in the middle of it.

You can over-analyse the cleaning. The reason it seems so important is that Huntington's drags you in the direction of chaos. Life is less ordered. Accidents, spillages, outbursts, upsets are just below the surface, waiting to happen. You can't do much about that. But you can create as much order and spick and span-ness as possible around the person with HD as a kind of symbolic buffer, a circle of calm. You can't do anything about the chaotic thinking and unpredictability. But you can try for a Zen garden effect on the kitchen and the living room. As long as you're prepared to do it all again every ten minutes.

The alternative is that the person with HD ends up surrounded by a mess that accumulates at a superhuman rate, oblivious to it themselves. Being dishevelled is a sign of not being cared for. Being surrounded by mess speaks of the same thing.

So, the never-ending mopping up of spilt coffee, scraping of lasagne off the carpet, emptying of ashtrays, changing of food-spattered clothes, making sure there are enough clean clothes for Sandy to change into, and, yes, mopping of strawberry milkshake from the ceiling, is a constant and recurring act of love, or at least compassion. The mess becomes a symptom or a manifestation of the illness. Fighting back the mess becomes one of the few tangible things you can do to combat it.

BH or Before Huntington's

What can I say about us before Huntington's Disease was in our midst? It seems such a long time ago, somebody else's life, dimly remembered. When we met in London in our early twenties, Sandy and I seemed to complement each other – the old yin–yang cliché. She had been a journalist, had got married, had a young child and was going back to college to get a degree. I had gone from a state school to Cambridge, where I had developed a large chip on my shoulder in resentment at the privileged, often not very bright private school types I was surrounded with there. After my degree I'd fled to Paris for a year to put off having to get a job. Then I came back to England wanting to become a journalist.

I was broke, teaching English to foreign students and living back in my parents' house when I first met Sandy. My mum was a childminder and Sandy used to drop Bromley at our house in the morning on her way to college. Sand later turned this into a joke that she used when telling people how we met. Our local authority, Hammersmith Council, was amazing, she would tell people. Not only did they find you a childminder, they threw in a new husband for free.

Journalism was our initial common ground. The complementary parts to us, the edges where we seemed to fit together well, were that I was the worrier, the glass-half-empty type, whereas she seemed serene and unbothered, as if she had a calm pool at her centre. I found this intriguing. She helped cancel out my mildly pessimistic way of looking at everything. We also shared a sense of humour and had a similar set of values. We felt that a lot of what people aspired to, particularly materially, was absurd. We both had a sense of being outsiders or non-conformists. Sandy in particular likes to see herself as a rebel. We both wanted a life lived by choice, not by convention.

Sandy, having been a fashion journalist, looked particularly unconventional – blonde, spiked hair and a self-assembled collection of budget clothing that always fell together to form something extraordinary. People turned to look in the street. Her friends were always trying to copy her sense of style, but never quite got there.

I remember a few years later working together on a writing job with Sandy. We were at the BBC Good Food Show, writing a show newspaper for the organizers of the event. As we left our hotel that morning, we passed in the lobby Karen Franklin, the fashion journalist who used to front a BBC TV programme called *The Clothes Show*. She was checking in at reception, as the annual Clothes Show event was on at the same venue as the event we were working at, but the following week.

Out of the corner of her eye, Karen Franklin spotted Sandy and me approaching the desk. She stopped signing in and turned to stare at Sandy, pen still in hand. She described a 360 degree circle, turning slowly on the spot as she followed our progress out through the lobby and to our car. You could see the 'Wow!' in her eyes. She was mentally taking notes. I couldn't understand what Sandy did with a few chains, bangles and dangly earrings that turned dressing into an art form, but it was obviously a talent that even the fashionistas recognized. *Is*, I should say, not was. I've included that anecdote as an example of Sandy's unconventional approach to how she presents herself in public. She tends to make an impression. In fact, she enjoys it.

So, I was impressed by her style as well as her substance. Things didn't run entirely smoothly, however. Sandy came with a child attached and a marriage. But the marriage was collapsing, by all accounts, and Bromley was an easy-to-love child. She and I fell in love, started a life together, and committed to sharing everything – both of us going out to work, taking it in turns to drop Brom at school, cook, wash up, clean, pay the bills and so on. We did the usual things a young family does – moved into a flat, got a mortgage, worked on our careers, spent the weekends taking Brom out to kids' theatres, to Chinatown in central London for dim sum, and to play football on Hampstead Heath.

The second half of our twenties and the first half of our thirties were happy times, I seem to remember – though this does feel,

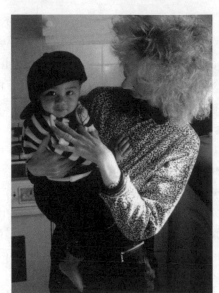

Sandy with Danny, 1992. It's all your fault, Dan. Love Dad.

oddly, like someone else's memories. (It's as if we are not the same people now which, in many ways, we are not. Huntington's does that to you.) We had a shared and close group of friends. We went to the pub, had people over for dinner and Sunday afternoon pop quizzes, took Brom to parties where our friends all wanted to talk to him and ignored us because he was the coolest six-year-old in the world. Sandy and I were even in a rock band together for a few years, playing gigs in clubs around London. We were happy. Not all the time. But mostly. We felt normal, in a non-conformist, slightly rebellious way, of course.

A slow unravelling

I can chart our apparent decline as a couple almost from the moment Danny was born. Sorry, Dan, if you are reading this. I'm not trying to lay that at your door. It's just a coincidence that you came along at that time. Actually, if it inspires enough guilt in you to get you to do more chores around the house to help me out then, yes, it is all your fault.

Like your brother, you were and are a very-loved child. That happiness at your arrival masked the fact that your mum seemed to take a long time to recover from your birth. We were still a happy family. But, the first signs of fraying started to appear around the edges. Tensions started gradually, almost imperceptibly, to emerge.

Sandy seemed exhausted and distracted in the months after Danny was born, finding it hard to get back into the groove of work again and apparently unwilling or unable – I'm now not sure which – to ease back into the role of partner. That's what we had always been, partners. We never regained that. Instead, I began to stretch to fill parental, work and domestic responsibilities that we used to share, but that Sandy seemed temporarily unable to deal with. As time dragged on, the 'temporarily' became more permanent.

I found myself making more family decisions on my own and taking on more tasks that used to be shared, because they simply weren't being done. I became increasingly resentful and a nag. The pattern of our conversations changed, from sharing thoughts, ideas and feelings to me complaining that something hadn't been done (maybe dinner cooked or the bathroom cleaned if it was her turn to do one or the other) and Sandy responding with a series of defensive one-liners that became predictable after a while. The one I remember most clearly is 'If it's that important to you, do it yourself.' She often seemed exhausted and distracted.

Something crept into the tone of our conversations that had never been there before. It felt at best like a loss of respect, at worst a kind of low-level contempt.

Never lose sight of how lucky you are

Before this chapter gets too bleak, I just want to say that things are better now than they were then. Every good day we have, and we have a lot of them, makes me think how lucky we are. Half the world's population live on less than $2 a day. We are luckier and better off, in terms of learning, leisure opportunities, living conditions, support services, than at a rough guess 90 per cent of people who ever lived. Yes, even with the Huntington's Disease in the family.

I came across this account of a woman with Huntington's the other day on a website. It was a painful reminder of how much worse things could be. Her name was Sarah:

> Everywhere she went children would taunt her, thinking she was drunk, and try to mimic her walk. She was frequently roughed up as she travelled back and forth…waiting for buses.
>
> One day she came home all roughed up, bruised and without her purse. She was hysterical and claimed that she had been raped.
>
> Sarah's nephew, Jack Kressly, took…her to Passavant Hospital. Jack hoped that they would diagnose her once and for all, and prescribe treatment.
>
> She was examined by the proper specialists, and they concluded that she had the usual symptoms for Huntington's Disease: choreic movements, flailing arms, jerking head, poor speech, unsteady gait. They also concluded that she had paranoid tendencies.
>
> However, during her stay, a careless physician took it upon himself to give a demonstration of her HD symptoms in the auditorium for the benefit of other doctors. He had her try to walk a straight line, held up her arm as it moved about, and pointed out her head movements. He also questioned her about her condition.
>
> Sarah became hysterical. She understood only too well the ramifications of the demonstration. (Kressly 1995)

Sometimes you read about a person who has Huntington's Disease, particularly if they are coping with it on their own and it's undiagnosed, and your heart goes out to them. Sarah's story, above, for example, moved me enormously when I came across it on a website where people have shared their experiences of Hunting-ton's Disease. What made it so moving was that I could easily imagine my wife in that situation.

It is then that you realize how lucky we are to have a loving, sup-portive network around Sandy. Because you get a graphic insight into what could happen without it.

I want to stress this point now, that we are lucky and life is good, because sections of this chapter may give the impression that all is doom and despair. It's not. It starts out that way when you discover the illness is in the family (and, in our case, before finding out, when the illness was affecting our lives but we weren't aware that it was). And you of course have down periods when you struggle, even in the midst of good ones. But there is always a way forward.

Difficult times

Around the time of Danny's birth, Sandy's dad came back into her life after a long absence, a significant change which she found increasingly traumatic. It turned out he was ill, though it took a while and at least one false diagnosis before we discovered it was Huntington's Disease.

With Sandy's brother and sister we then became involved in a protracted and painful time that lasted a few years. As he became increasingly mentally and physically ill, Sandy and her brother and sister had to intervene to help their dad more. They had decided between them not to tell their mum that Brian had reappeared in their lives. She had endured years of exhausting aggression and pain during her marriage and they did not want to plunge her back into a past that she was still recovering from.

One day I dropped Sandy off so she could clean up her dad's flat for him. He no longer seemed able to clean up himself. When I picked her up a couple of hours later she appeared shaken and couldn't talk. Her dad had told her there were people inside the TV talking to him. But one particular thing shook her the most. 'I had to clean shit off the walls,' she whispered to me later, when I finally persuaded her to tell me why she was so down.

Visiting him at the home a year or so later was difficult too, as Sandy, her sister Wendy and brother Geoff were seeing what they and their children might become. They were also having to cope with visiting a father who had acted terribly towards them and their mother.

And then he died, which seemed to plunge Sandy into a prolonged period of grief that even now she occasionally slips back into.

Dismantling the family

Over those five years, I stretched to help Sandy, as you do if your partner is going through a tough time. We drifted from being a two-income family to mostly, and eventually only, a one-income family. After a few years of this I started to feel the strain and tried handing a few responsibilities back to Sandy. Household budgeting, for example. It didn't work. We kept slipping into the red.

Looking back, it is baffling how your relationship can change so profoundly but so gradually that you do not notice it happening. It's like children growing up, I guess. One day you turn around and think, 'Who on earth is that enormous young man? Where's our little boy gone?' There was a gradual decline in our relationship, until I reached a level of despair without realizing it.

The actual circumstances that led to this state were what seemed to be the gradual loss of the person I thought I had known, loved and been married to, and an equally slow and parallel stripping away of my sense of self and what I was for. It was as if the Huntington's Disease, which was at that time living with us but without us knowing it was there, was slowly dismantling us as a family. We did recover from this later, but you need to know that this is where I think we bottomed out as a family. That's as bad as it's been so far. They were dark times.

The house seemed full of constant anger, dissatisfaction with each other, frustration and sadness. There were claims and counter-claims of violence between Sandy and myself, threats of the police being called, solicitors' letters sent from one party to the other full of unrecognizable accusations. The anger in the house was at times so huge it exploded. One particularly bad night I remember as being possibly the lowest point. It was about two in the morning. Everything that could be smashed was being smashed. Glasses, plates, bowls, ashtrays, vases, ornaments, family pictures pulled from the walls, glass jugs – all were being systematically smashed one by one, with a carpet of glass and broken crockery spreading across the kitchen floor.

Along with the smashing sounds, I remember a great screaming – a howl of rage and despair coming from my wife – and a scared little boy in his pyjamas peering over the balcony from upstairs, shouting, 'What's wrong? What's happening?'

'Go back to bed, I'm dealing with it. It'll be OK,' I shouted up distractedly. The tone of my voice was so fraught it can't have sounded reassuring. I didn't in fact have a clue what to do.

He doesn't seem to recall it now, but for several years after that horrible night Danny, our younger son, would become very anxious and watchful and quiet – the 'quiet' being particularly unusual for him – at the slightest hint of tension between his mum and me, especially in the evenings. I think what he was scared of after that night was the prospect that any hint of friction between us might escalate into another long night of horrors.

Danny also made an association in his head from then onwards, I think, between alcohol and aggressive behaviour. He became very anti-drink. And he took responsibility for trying to improve the atmosphere, as children often do. For years afterwards he had a habit of sticking his head into whatever room I was in and saying, with a cheerful grin 'You all right?' I'd then hear him do the same elsewhere in the house, wherever his mum was.

You realize how bad you've let things become when your kids feel they regularly have to check on your state of mind and well-being instead of the other way round. I should insert a reminder here that although we knew Sandy's dad had died of Huntington's Disease at this stage, we did not know we were living with it ourselves. I assumed we were living with an outpouring of grief at the death of a parent, but couldn't understand why the anger that accompanied it was mostly directed at me, and why it was lasting for so long.

You stopped being happy

There didn't seem a lot of love left in our family at this time. Bromley and I were increasingly at loggerheads, just as his mum and I were. You can often lose sight of the downward spiral a family falls into, but it was Brom who gave me a flash of insight into it. He was in his late teens and dealing with some tough issues, including having to absorb into his life the information that he was at risk of inheriting a fatal illness. At that stage he had a one in four chance of inheriting the illness that had killed his granddad, while his mum had a one in two chance. He'd gone off the rails a bit. I think I would have done at his age, too.

I locked him and myself in the office I was renting at the time and said, 'Right, we're not leaving till we've had a proper conversation and got to the bottom of what is wrong.' Like most parents with teenagers who aren't following the rules, what I meant was 'What is wrong with *you?*' After about an hour of flailing around and getting nowhere, as you'd expect from two males trying to get to the bottom of their emotions, Brom took me by surprise.

'You were doing so well at school, at home, everything. What's changed over the past couple of years? What's gone wrong?' I kept repeating. Brom was as confused as me. 'Just tell me one thing that's changed,' I finally said, to try and narrow the problem down. 'Well, *you* stopped being happy, for a start,' Brom blurted out, catching himself by surprise as much as me, I think.

And there's the rub. Kids are like lightning rods. Just because they're acting out and acting up doesn't mean the root of the problem is necessarily in them to be fixed. Often they're channelling family emotions. Maybe a better image is that they are holding up a mirror to tell you something about your own behaviour, even if it's being done sub-consciously. If you want your kids to be happy and secure, you have to be so yourself. Partly because it shows them there's nothing to worry about. And partly because it shows them that there's nothing going on that's their fault. I hadn't realized that. Just as I hadn't realized I'd stopped being happy until Brom told me.

'You're the problem, not me'

I think we need a few paragraphs here to explain some of the tension that develops within a family that has Huntington's.

What's the strongest force in the universe? Love? Hate? Gravity? Compound interest, as Einstein supposedly once answered? No, it's none of these. The strongest force in the universe is Denial. With Huntington's, Denial tends to come with a capital 'D'.

When you develop the symptoms of Huntington's, all the things you used to be able to do, from work to keeping control of the household budget, gradually slip away from you, ever so gradually. A natural reaction to this, I discovered later, is to externalize the problem. If you know you are at risk of inheriting a terminal illness and have chosen not to take the test that tells you if you have the gene, then when things start to go wrong in your life, Denial can take over.

You can't look inside for the causes of your increasing difficulties in interacting with the world because the most obvious answer is the most unbearable. So, it is common to project the causes outwards on to the nearest person. I've shared notes with other people who have a spouse with HD, one of whom told me:

> I used to be mystified by the accusations he would suddenly shout at me, like 'All you do is watch television,' or 'You're so boring, you never do anything!' or 'You never help anyone with anything. You live a completely selfish life!' I hardly ever sit down, yet he's always watching the TV. I used to be hurt and indignant, as he seemed to be describing himself, not me. Then it hit me recently that he was doing exactly that, projecting on to me the things about his own life that he found so frustrating. He didn't want to be that person.

Equally, it can be easy for the spouse to accept this role as being the cause of all the problems that the Huntington's Disease is actually causing. So, not only do you live with a lot of the fallout of this disease, you become the scapegoat. I remember Maggie, Sandy's mum, telling me how her confidence and sense of self were eroded over the years by constantly being told that everything that went wrong, from her husband Brian losing his job (which happened many times) to his constant affairs, was somehow all her fault.

Giving up

If your partner isn't happy and you are constantly being told it's your fault, you might eventually believe it, try and change maybe, and if that fails, give up. Or your confidence gets crushed as you accept the blame for everything that's not working. Watch out for that one, by the way. So, that's a pattern lots of families with HD go through.

In our case, whenever we got into an argument, which was frequently, Sandy's refrain had become 'You're the problem. You are why I am so unhappy. Just leave me alone.' After several years of this I began to believe it to some extent and removed myself. We told

Brom, who was almost 17, that I wasn't leaving him and his brother Dan, who was then six; that I was still their dad, but their mum and I needed a trial separation. We didn't tell Dan anything, as the plan was that I would turn up at the house early in the morning, before he got up, take him to school and be there after work in the evening, till he went to bed. So I naively hoped he wouldn't notice.

But, looking back, I don't think saying, 'I'm not leaving you' to kids does any good. When one parent leaves the family home, they always think it is them you are leaving.

I rented a room in town, four miles away, and became a reverse commuter of sorts, coming back to the village for the day, working in an office I rented there, heading home to see the boys and then leaving in the evenings. During the six months I lived away from the house, my life moved on. I started to see a possible new life for me. Over that six months, with the help of people who loved and valued me, I fixed myself a bit. Not completely, but I had been lifted up off the bottom. And I'd come to the conclusion there was no way forward at home. Sandy and I were heading towards a divorce.

Your wife has Huntington's Disease

Then I received a letter. The letter was from our genetics counsellor, asking me to come in and see her. We'd had genetic counselling as a family a few times after we had found out that Sandy was 50 per cent at risk of inheriting the illness that killed her father, and that the boys were therefore each 25 per cent at risk. If Sandy turned out to have the gene, the boys would move up to 50 per cent at risk, as if on a moving staircase with no stop button.

Genetics counsellors help families deal with having your world turned upside down, which is what happens when you are told you have an inherited and incurable illness in the family. So, I went to see what Ivana, the counsellor, had to say. I sat down in the chair opposite her. In between us, on a coffee table, was the usual box of tissues that I remembered from previous visits. It seemed to be an essential part of the counsellor's toolbox. I guess a lot of tears got shed in that room.

'I've asked you here because I understand that you and Sandy are living apart now,' began Ivana. 'Er, that's right,' I said, puzzled. Then it was all over in a few seconds: 'Well, I thought you should know, as you are making decisions that affect your whole family, that in my opinion, Sandy definitely has Huntington's Disease.'

There was a pause. Ivana seemed to be waiting for a reaction. I didn't seem to have any available. So, she carried on: 'I know she hasn't had the test to determine for sure that she has the gene. But, all I can say is that I have seen enough people with Huntington's, and seen enough of Sandy, to be able to say that I'm as sure as I can be that she has the illness.'

Of course, I had known deep down. What's the most powerful force in the universe, again? Yes, I had succumbed over the years to Denial with a big D myself. When you are 50 per cent at risk of inheriting the illness, you try and make yourself be positive and not interpret every dropped coffee cup as an early warning sign. Similarly, the people around you train themselves to be positive and not to share concerns with each other that maybe the symptoms are showing and a person at risk does indeed have the gene, because this kind of worry seems disloyal, an abandonment of the facade of sunny optimism we all try and keep going like a fixed grin that has become a grimace. I made a last ditch, feeble attempt to fend off the inevitable: 'What makes you so certain?' I remember asking. 'You could be wrong, surely.'

'The way she walks, the depression, sudden changes of mood, but mostly the movements...' Ivana tailed off. Clearly, I had to go home. Inside, I felt a cry of protest from a small, selfish voice. It was the part of me that had made a dash for freedom and felt it was being pulled back at the last minute, like Steve McQueen on his motorbike in *The Great Escape*; almost clear, but unable to make that last leap and ending up stuck in the barbed wire.

The more selfless part of me realized I had a big job to do now and doubted very much that I was up to it. I looked away out of the window.

'Do you want a tissue?' asked Ivana.

Coming home

Family break-ups are common when HD is changing the behaviour of one member of the family and the others don't know what is happening. I suspect what I had been doing when I had left the family home, at some kind of sub-conscious level, was running while I had the chance; while the causes of our break-up could be put down to mutual incompatibility, before someone told me other-wise. Then Ivana the counsellor broke the spell by telling me what, deep down, I knew already. I had no choice but to go back home. The vow was 'in sickness and in health' after all. The incompatibil-ity of the previous years made far more sense now. I had begun a different life in the six months we were apart, one with a prospect of some happiness for me at least. But I now had to end that life and go back.

Even so, I had no confidence at all that I would be strong enough to deal with the situation at home. I'd seen Sandy's dad's decline from Huntington's and had heard the family war stories about the havoc the illness had wreaked when Sandy was growing up. Extreme unreasonable behaviour, constant arguments, bullying, drinking, affairs, lost jobs, money problems, spousal abuse, the kids being treated badly... Sandy's mum had eventually given up and divorced their dad. But the difference between that situation and ours now, which must have made it so much harder for Sandy's mother, was that no one knew then it was the Huntington's that was causing that kind of behaviour.

Well, probably. I guess you should add 'probably' here because one thing that is always impossible to separate out definitively when you look back is which part of someone's behaviour was caused by the illness and which part was something they would have done anyway. We never really know for sure.

Anyway, I came home, we patched things up and life gradually…I was about to say got back to normal, but there is no 'normal' to go back to once you find out HD is definitely in the family. We learnt, over time, to create a new kind of 'normal' is what I mean, one that is infinitely better than the strained, angry atmosphere that tended to be around when we didn't know that HD was living with us in the house. It did take a long time, though. For the first three years there was a big roadblock to any attempts to move forward and create a better understanding within the family. Because, as well as having to rebuild trust with Sandy and Bromley, an inevitable phase when a family comes back together, there was a secret problem I was unable to share.

Two different realities

Although I knew Sandy had HD, she didn't. She had decided in the past not to have the test that would tell her if she had the gene (and hence if she would get the disease). 'If it turned out I had the gene, I wouldn't be able to bear it. I'd rather not know,' she said on several occasions. After I came back to live at home, every couple of months I would remind her that she had always said this – that knowing she had the gene would be too much to bear – and asked her if she still felt that way. The answer was always 'Definitely, yes.'

A higher percentage of people who know they have the HD gene commit suicide than the average population. So, when someone at risk says 'I couldn't bear it if it turned out I had the gene,' you tend to interpret that the worst possible way. For three years after I came back home to the family house, I lived with Sandy knowing she had not just the gene but the symptoms, while she didn't want to know. So I didn't tell her.

In case you are wondering, it is possible to have symptoms and not notice them yourself. When you have HD, your mind can do some kind of double-take if it, for example, notices your right hand flying past the corner of your vision in a jerky movement that it didn't instruct the arm to do. Either your mind will ignore it, or part of your brain might take over and turn the movement into something else. Apparently this is called a 'pseudo-purposive movement'. I've seen someone with HD jerk forward in their seat (the involuntary movement), get up (the brain interpreting the move and turning it into what it thinks the person wants to do), turn around in a full circle, and sit back down again, all in one quite fluid movement. 'Are we going?' his wife asked. 'What do you mean?' he said. 'You just got up and sat back down,' she said. 'No, I didn't,' he said.

You can imagine how confused and flabbergasted I was after three pretty much exhausting years of carrying this information around and having to keep it from her, when Sandy found out by accident that she had the symptoms of HD. It wasn't her finding out that was flabbergasting. It was her reaction. After the initial shock had died down, she said it was a relief to finally know. So, I guess we could have told her three years earlier instead of the rest of the family keeping it a secret and scrambling to cover up the truth whenever it looked about to leak out. Somebody up there certainly has a strange sense of humour.

The power of acceptance

When you find you are living with something awful and powerful at the heart of your family and this awful thing is persistent and can't be beaten, you have a choice. You can feel sorry for yourselves and get mired in a 'poor me, why us?' mental ghetto. Or you accept it, gradually learn how to manage it, and get on with it. Acceptance takes time, years sometimes.

I heard one of the oldest surviving British soldiers from World War I on the radio the other day, just before he died aged an astonishing 110 or something like that. The interviewer asked him what the secret was of a long and happy life. He answered, 'Acceptance. Some things you just can't change. Accept them.' I imagine he was thinking of all the loved ones and friends he had lost along the way. In which case I think he meant, in particular, acceptance of loss. You can't live your life in mourning for what you had, or for what would have happened if your life had carried on as it was pre-Huntington's.

The 'Poor me, why us' feeling comes from a lack of real acceptance; from a sense that there is some other life you should be living (or were living, in fact) – a better life free from this affliction – and you will continue to mourn the absence of that better life and feel sorry for yourself. Maybe you keep that sorrow hidden or you share it with anyone who will listen. It's a natural first stage you go through when you are told you have Huntington's Disease in the family. But it's a stage you have to learn to move on from if you are to triumph in any way over the disease. There's a paradox here, in that you need to embrace the loss and accept it to then be able to move on and beat it.

What do I mean by 'beat it'? I mean live life to the full and be creative in helping the person with HD and the family members at risk from it to live life to the full themselves. I mean refusing to feel cowed and scared all the time. If Huntington's is ultimately life-diminishing, then you set out to ensure the family members who have it and are at risk of it – and you, yourself if you are not at risk but the people you love are – live the fullest lives possible.

Seize the day: living in the moment

Being able to live in the moment is Huntington's greatest gift. That is bound to sound odd. But, let me explain. You don't have to be a starry-eyed optimist to feel like this. I certainly am not. But after you've finished grieving for your lost future (which can take years), you realize that the imagined future you are grieving for was never real anyway. Huntington's shocks you into an appreciation that all

we have, really, is 'now'. Your plans, even your subconscious ones, aren't your life. Moments are your life.

There is an odd intensity in our lives now, a kind of urge to appreciate those moments fully, savouring every good moment that happens. When life is likely to be snatched away at any moment, or at least shortened, there is a renewed vibrancy to it. Your capacity to enjoy it is enhanced. Instead of always planning for the future, you live for the moment. This is an age of hurry in which we are always being told we need to slow down, to stop and smell the coffee. Or is it the flowers? Whatever. By taking you outside of the main, fast-flowing current of life that most other people seem stuck in, Huntington's actually gives you the perspective you need to slow down and appreciate life.

With any illness that involves a gradual decline you learn to appreciate every enjoyable moment that comes along. You also learn that you need to manufacture some of those moments. I learnt that from Sandy's mum, who used to arrange family picnics and outings that brought her grandchildren together whenever she could. She told me once she did it to create strong, enjoyable family memories for the children in particular to draw on later in life.

So many people live humdrum lives working in jobs they do not find inspiring, waiting for some retirement date when they can do what they want to do, rather than what they have to do. Then, when that moment comes, millions of people look back and think, 'What on earth was I doing? Was that my life?' Not us. We now have a reckless streak in the family, a kind of wanton readiness to enjoy the moment. Because we know that's all that any of us have.

The danger here, of course, is veering into an extreme of hedonism or nihilism. Not having a positive sense of a better future that you are pushing towards can lead to that 'What's the point of anything' malaise that drifts you into depression. It is easy to slip into the idea that living for the moment means a life of excess and focusing only on your own needs. The constant drinking and affairs

that happen with some people who have HD may partly be down to that sense that there is no future so the rules don't apply to you any more. More often they are down to the disinhibition – the removal of the self-monitoring that stops us doing things that aren't good for us or are hurtful to those around us – that is a symptom of Huntington's.

Anyway, that reckless streak I was talking about. Here's an example...

I'll have the Mustang convertible, please

Sandy loves detective stories. A series of whodunnit novels she loves are set on the Maine coast of New England. The books sparked off in her a powerful desire to see the rough beauty of that coastline for real. So, we went, on a whim. I'm a freelance, so there is some elasticity in how much I earn. If I want more money, I work harder and longer hours. Then we blow it all on travelling to distant places and I start all over again. We go to places we would have put off till future years if Huntington's hadn't been in the family.

That's how we ended up in the Hertz car rental office at Boston airport, from where we were due to drive up the coast to Maine. My eyes strayed from the mid-sized compact on the rentals chart to the Mustang convertible, with a button on the dashboard that you press to make the car roof appear or disappear. 'How much to rent that one?' I asked. 'A thousand dollars,' said the rental guy, chewing his gum and grinning, with a 'Dare you' glint in his eye. 'We'll have that instead of the mid-size,' I said without missing a beat. Don't get me wrong. We're not rampant materialists who crave fast cars and mansions. I just felt the need to break out, to thumb my nose at the restrictions that HD tries to coil around you and that constrict your choices in life.

I wondered if it was really my voice saying it. And I was unable to stop the mental calculator in the dim recesses of my brain starting up. How much extra freelance work would I need to say 'yes' to over

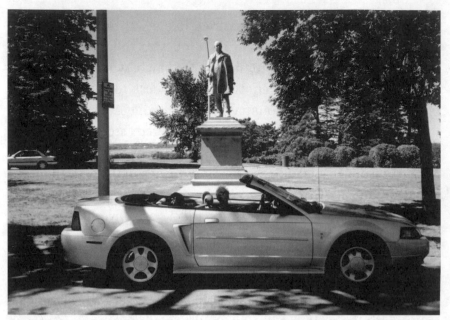

Sandy (front passenger seat), Danny (just about visible, doing a V-sign in the back seat) both dwarfed by an enormous Mustang Convertible, Portland, Maine. The guy on the plinth wouldn't stop staring at the car.

the next few weeks to pay for this impulsive decision, is what it was trying to calculate. And exactly which hours of the night or weekend could that work be shoe-horned into? I'm sure I heard something snap as the calculator gave up.

There's a reorganization of your brain that goes on in the background, like a frantic Rubik's cube re-alignment to try and re-set the colours, to absorb decisions like this without your head exploding. It's accompanied by a vertigo-like feeling of having made a decision that will help push your family over the edge into a slow slide into the financial mess that many HD families end up in. You ground yourself by just making a mental note that you won't allow that to happen, and you'll figure it out when you get home.

You end up doing mad things like this on a whim: 'What the hell,' says a voice somewhere in your head; 'Life is short; Sand's life will be shorter than most; just do it now while she can enjoy it.' It

doesn't have to be expensive luxuries, like it was on this occasion. Plenty of times we haven't had the money to follow a whim like that. It could just be going to the pub for lunch, which Sandy loves doing, and leaving the urgent work on the desk for a while, or just going for a drive in the country.

So, on this occasion, Sandy was chauffeured through the coastal towns of New England in a slow, winding cruise, in a silver Mustang Convertible with the top down, her spiky blonde hair just about poking imperiously out of the top on the passenger's side (those cars are enormous and she's a little over five foot tall) and attracting admiring glances from the American car-loving public.

Which made a nice change from the surreptitious glances, or mouth-gaping stares, from people wondering what's wrong with the small blonde woman that makes her walk in such a jerky, apparently comical way. It was like one of those 'queen for a day' things. Yes, and I didn't mind driving it, either.

Some people stare

Well, it's natural, I suppose. But it's intensely annoying to be stared at when we are out and about as a family. We, the boys and me, try and take our cue from Sandy, who appears blissfully unaware of being such a head-turner. But it's not always easy to ignore when people are being particularly rude. I've read the other draft chapters in this book (cheating, I know) and I notice Brom, Dan and Chan all mention this, too, so it's clearly something that makes us all angry.

Thoughtful people might look our way in surprise, then quickly stop looking when they realize this isn't a drunk person in the middle of the day attracting their attention, but someone with an illness. Less thoughtful people continue to gawp, or even nudge each other or change their position to get a better look. These are the ones I used to target for retribution. It's bad enough having a terminal illness without some people seeming to find it a spectator sport.

I developed a way of dealing with them without bothering Sandy. In the supermarket, for example, I would let her forge ahead, charging through the aisles and scattering the crowd ahead of her as she tends to do. One of the symptoms of Huntington's is a loss of sense of personal space and of self-consciousness. This can be very useful in a supermarket. If Sandy sees something she wants and people are in the way, she's not going to wait politely or weave her way between them. She barrels forward and it's like Moses parting the waves. The other shoppers just fall away on either side.

I cruise along behind her, pushing the shopping cart, keeping an eye out for anyone who takes offence or is paying Sandy too much attention. Then I slide in between them and, if necessary, have a quiet word. I have stopped doing it now, though, as I think I was getting a bit mean in biting back. One particular incident I remember was the last time I had a go at anyone in public for being rude behind Sandy's back. We were in the supermarket. Sandy was a few yards ahead of me and had stopped in front of a shelf of soap powder. She was shuffling forward, lining herself up to lunge for the shelf, which was quite high and awkward for her to reach.

In between her and me were an elderly couple, early seventies maybe, sharing the pushing of their own shopping cart. The husband seemed captivated by Sandy's attempts to reach the shelf. He nudged his wife with his elbow, pointed at Sandy and began to imitate her shuffle, laughing at his wife as he did it.

Having no blunt instrument to hand, I considered a sharp blow to the ankles with my own shopping cart as the quickest option, but went for the jugular instead. I eased around the couple and slowed down as I passed him, as if this was a drive-by shooting. In a way, it was. I paused just long enough to say, in a voice too low for Sandy to hear, the killer lines: 'Glad you find my wife's terminal illness so funny. Don't you think it's bad enough not being able to get your muscles to work properly without some people being amused by it?'

I looked back. They'd stopped and he had a look of horror on his face. 'But, I didn't…I wouldn't…I mean, if I'd known…', he stammered.

OK, so it needs doing sometimes. Those who stare or mock need educating about how wearying it is for people who look different to be constantly stared at and have people whispering about them in public. But the look of horror on the old man's face made me feel I'd set him up and then knocked him down. It had started off feeling the right thing to do. It ended up feeling mean.

Where does strength come from?

When a friend or my mum or someone asks, 'How are things going?' I'm always reminded of the joke about the man who falls from the top of the Empire State Building. Every floor he passes, people hear him saying to himself, 'So far, so good.' With Huntington's you always feel something big is looming, that we are heading towards the pavement, albeit more slowly than from the top of the Empire State Building. But, aren't we all? That's what life is. We're all heading towards an end. It's making the most of the fall that counts.

I don't mean this to sound sentimental but any strength I have in this situation comes from being constantly inspired by Sandy, Sandy's mum, Brom, Dan and Chan – the people most immediately affected by having HD in our family – and wanting to do the best for them and not let them down. It's no exaggeration to say I watch them in a kind of state of wonder as they go about their daily lives.

When you see and hear people you care for laughing, teasing each other, being creative, arguing animatedly but good naturedly, working hard at something and getting the results they need to move their life forwards – *despite* this horrible thing hanging over us or, more accurately, in the middle of us – then it makes me feel I have no right to be scared or exhausted in the face of Huntington's Disease.

If Brom and Dan can get up every morning and live their lives with their characteristic optimism, cheeriness and amazing generosity of spirit, like they do, when they are at risk of inheriting it and I'm not, then who the hell am I to allow myself to get down or, in the worst case scenario, panic? They, Sand, Chan, and Sand's mum inspire me to raise my game, making me feel that line Jack Nicholson comes out with in the film *As Good As It Gets* (I know, I know, another pop culture reference – like I said, I don't get out much, and if you have trouble sleeping, you end up watching a lot of DVDs…).

'You make me want to be a better man,' he said.

If you were the one with HD

I try to think myself into Sandy's situation sometimes. And it is that process that is humbling, really. Imagine waking up and, for a second, not being conscious of HD, then having it flood back into your mind, like the dawning awareness that it is, in fact, Monday and time to go to work, not, as you had thought while you were drifting into consciousness, Saturday and time to turn over and fall asleep again. Magnify that feeling of heartsink a million times – knowing, again, that you are starting a day with a terminal illness hanging over you.

Now imagine waking up with that knowledge and still being able to jump up – or, increasingly, stagger up (but with a determined sense of purpose) and greet the day with a loud 'Good morning!', like Sandy does. If it was me, I suspect I'd be curling up under the duvet and willing the world to go away. So, even the way Sandy gets up and faces Huntington's every day with a 'get out of my way' defiant attitude has always impressed me.

Sandy has a piece of body language that she uses to focus her energies. She'll be standing in the middle of the room and will suddenly clap her hands together once in a 'Right! Let's tackle this' kind of action, preparatory to launching herself forward into whatever she is about to do.

If you have HD your body will often just stop in the middle of what you are doing. You'll be walking along, or lurching with an unsteady gait, and will suddenly stop. This can lead to a comical pile up behind and people veering to one side to avoid you. It must be immensely frustrating to have to concentrate hard and clap your hands together to refocus your body on what you want to do, just as Dorothy's clicking together of the heels on her red shoes summoned the magic to get her where she wanted to go.

I admire Sandy's will to push on like that immensely, even if it's just to get from one side of the kitchen to the other and reach the coffee she is desperate for first thing in the morning. The human spirit, that thing that shouts from inside, 'Get up. Push on. Smile,' is inspiring, even if it's just driving you on to get down the stairs to the coffee and a cigarette in the morning, rather than to pull yourself up the last few steps to the top of the mountain to plant your flag.

What it means to be happy

Yes, I'm scared of what might happen to our boys, that one or both of them might inherit this illness. Yes, I carry around deep down a sense of loss and sadness. Yes, I am sometimes extremely tired. It is then that things always seem worse, that I feel least capable of keeping up with the progression of the illness in Sandy and am afraid it will overwhelm my ability to keep us going. But, there is far more to my life than that. I laugh. I enjoy my work. I love the company of my family and, when I can get my act together to see them, my friends. I put the kitchen stereo on loud and dance in the kitchen on Friday nights when I'm cooking (not a pretty sight).

I was reading about comparative happiness the other day. A survey reported in the newspaper found that, above a minimum required for the basics of life, it doesn't matter how much you earn. If you have a BMW on your drive but all your neighbours have a Porsche, you will be unhappy. Einstein was right. Everything's

relative. Well, what a crock of, er, rubbish it is to measure your own happiness like that, don't you think?

We all struggle to distance ourselves from that kind of comparison, but it's difficult, isn't it? Huntington's helps. It forces you to focus on what really counts. Some things that made me happy lately are: a surprise video message from Brom and Chan, singing 'Happy Birthday', that appeared on my phone; the sound of Dan laughing and joking with his friends, heard through the open home-office window as he walked up the front steps to the house after school; and Sandy shouting (volume control fails sometimes, remember) to her 11-year-old niece the other day, 'Bye Charis! Drive carefully!' as Charis and her mum got into the car to go home after a visit. We all collapsed laughing at that one, actually.

Our boys are driven, have an edge, an appetite for life. They want to do things young. Dan wants to write a book and goes at it with a passion. He'd written 70,000 words last count. Oh, he's just walked past my office door and shouted, '80,000 now'. This chapter is being written in real-time. Brom is starting businesses while he's still at college. A record company with his brilliant Canadian musician friend is his latest venture. Both the boys enjoy and appreciate their friends and life generally. They put nothing off, take nothing for granted. The strange gift that comes with this illness is that Huntington's Disease can make you realize what it means to be happy.

CHAPTER 7

A Cruel Inheritance: Brian's Story

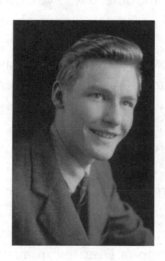

Brian Gibson, 25 May 1936 to 18 November 1995. Brian was a bright working class boy, a Geordie from the north-east of England. He became a trainee journalist and quickly rose through the ranks, first as a newspaper reporter before moving into TV. He was a TV news journalist, then a producer and editor of news and current affairs programmes at the BBC. He seems to have developed the symptoms of HD, which he inherited from his father, in his thirties. But it wasn't diagnosed till twenty years later. Two of his three children, myself and my brother, inherited the HD gene from him and have gone on to develop the disease.

Brian, my dad, died of pneumonia in a care home aged 59. This is a common cause of death for people with Huntington's Disease. My own chapter in this book, and my sister Wendy's chapter, plus the absence of a chapter from my mum who had such a terrible time in the later years of my dad's life, give the correct impression that the older Brian acted like a monster. In fact, I've seen that word used a few times in descriptions of Huntington's Disease – that it turns people into monsters – and I wince each time I see it.

There is a big question here about what the core of a person is. It's a question that is largely beyond me, but I wanted to put this chapter in this book as a reminder, at least in the first half of this chapter, of what my dad was like in the first half of his life, before Huntington's Disease changed how he behaved.

He didn't quite make it to 60. Since we know how Huntington's typically progresses, with the onset of symptoms arriving in your thirties or forties, we can divide his life pretty neatly into two halves. Up to 30 we can assume he was free of the symptoms of Huntington's Disease, and hence that the way he behaved then was the real man. The first half of this chapter reflects this. After 30, an age I've chosen simply because 1. it's the halfway point in his life and 2. we can be fairly certain Huntington's didn't make a significant appearance before then, he began behaving in the way that you will have picked up as 'monstrous' if you have read the other chapters of this book. That version of my dad, the Huntington's version, makes his appearance in the second half of this chapter.

There is a caveat I have to add here. Wendy, my sister, remembers stories showing that Brian did in fact have quite a temper when he was young. On one occasion he flew into a rage in a youth club and apparently put his hands through a glass window pane. He still had the scars on his arms as an adult.

Brian as he was

The dad I remember from my childhood was kind, loving, funny, creative, enthusiastic, passionate, slightly madcap, endlessly interested in everything, curious, articulate, charming and very clever. This is my recollection, I should emphasize. Perhaps I am the luckiest of the three of his children as I am the oldest. So I am more likely to remember him when he was more himself and less changed by the Huntington's Disease.

As my sister Wendy has pointed out in her chapter of this book, even though we know it was the HD that caused his violent behaviour later in life, it is hard for those who were there and experienced it to separate out the person from the illness. Forgiving a person for that kind of behaviour is hard enough. But, with HD you need to go even further and not just forgive the person but acknowledge that they don't actually need forgiving. They weren't responsible. It simply wasn't them.

Maybe it's easier to do that if you know at the time that the HD is the cause of the behaviour. If you only find out decades later often the emotional scars are so deep set they refuse to heal. Or they heal very slowly. The logic that says, 'It wasn't him, it was the illness' doesn't change your feelings towards that person instantly, if ever. You end up with conflicting emotions.

When my dad died, my brother and I put together a remembrance piece to be read out at his funeral. My sister was in the US at the time and so wasn't able to have any input in what was said. The remembrance piece leaves out any reference to his Huntington's-influenced behaviour in the second half of his life because we wanted to remember him as he was, himself. On reflection, I think this sanitized version of Dad that was presented at his funeral, a version that stripped out the Huntington's Disease, was largely at my urging.

Both Wendy and Geoff, but particularly Wendy (my brother was often away training and then at sea as part of his career as a

ship's engineer in the oil industry), had seen the worst of my dad's behaviour in the couple of years after I left home to go to college in London. In fact Wendy recently told me that it turned into a major problem for her that she hadn't had any input into his funeral. She was horrified at the end result of his remembrance piece and how 'perfect' he was made out to be. It actually caused her some trauma, which she had to take to a counsellor, because it was like he was trying to erase and mess with her memories even from the grave. When Dad had forced Wendy to meet him as a condition of continuing to pay maintenance so she could go to college, he spent most of those meetings denying he had ever done anything bad to our mum. So you can see why Wendy would be freaked by what I wrote. Sorry, Wend. This is the remembrance piece we read out:

> Brian will always be remembered by his family for his intelligence, campaigning journalism, talent – and the fact that he achieved so much in such a short space of time.
>
> He started out as a trainee reporter with the *Evening Chronicle* in 1952 before deciding he wanted to get into television. He applied for a post in the BBC's Newcastle upon Tyne studio and was given a reference by a friend and colleague Fred Billany, who said at the time that Brian was one of the most promising young journalists he had ever known.
>
> In just five years he became Head of News and Current Affairs for Tyne Tees Television, a post he also held at Yorkshire TV, at the age of just 32. But after clashes with his boss Donald Baverstock he resigned, not once but twice in one week, himself becoming the main story on the front page of the *Daily Mail* that week. A news man becoming the news story – that must have made him smile. I can just imagine him shouting, 'There are more important things to stick on

the front page, for crying out loud! Where's their news sense?'

Perhaps it was his work with the pioneering TV magazine programme *Nationwide*, where Dad was a founder producer, that gave him the most satisfaction. It allowed him to travel the country extensively, using his enquiring mind to dig out stories. Many of these focused on Northern Ireland. He was a regular visitor and always stayed in Belfast's Europa Hotel, which was notorious not for its service but because it was Northern Ireland's most-bombed hotel.

One of his prized possessions was his Europa Hotel tie, which was presented to all guests who stayed there and survived to tell the tale. In the mid-1970s he edited *Day & Night*, the first current affairs TV programme to centre on the work of the police.

Brian was the only journalist to sit through the entire trial of the Birmingham Six and it was from this experience that he wrote his book *The Birmingham Bombs*. Dad also wrote many unpublished novels and scripts.

Whatever he was working on he threw himself into with immense enthusiasm. Most nights his typewriter would clatter away into the small hours as he wrote his latest script or churned out yet another novel. His family soon learned to fall asleep to this strange background noise.

He will also be remembered as a man with a creative temperament to match his creative abilities. He once, in frustration, picked up his typewriter, opened the door and hurled it outside where it smashed to pieces on the patio.

On a personal level he was a very straightforward man – a Geordie by birth who never forgot his working class roots. He lacked bigotry and hated racism – people

of all colours and nationalities were welcomed into his home.

He loved his family and was in his element with young people, who responded to him naturally because of his interest in them and the fact that he treated them as adults. He despised snobbery and was never happier than when in his local Tandoori restaurant, with friends or family and a bottle of house red wine.

His children will remember him for the fact that he was more of a friend than a dad. He took a great interest in their lives but never interfered. He made it clear that he loved them for what they were and not what they achieved and was always there in a crisis.

One of his proudest moments was when he first became a granddad in 1981. He leaves behind him five grandchildren who will never know him properly. Perhaps some of them will inherit his charm and sense of humour. But he is best remembered for those early years of promise fulfilled and for the person he was then.

Dad's childhood

Hmmmm. Well, perhaps some of them will turn out to have inherited his charm and sense of humour. But, obviously, there are limits to what we want them to have inherited. What we didn't mention in that eulogy, which I guess is what that was, was anything about Dad's family or much about his childhood. In fact, I guess we skirted around a lot.

My father was one of four children. It would turn out decades later that he was the only one of the four to have inherited the faulty gene that leads to Huntington's Disease. God's dice fell right for the other three. Or God's coin toss, as it's a 50–50 chance for each person. But none of the family then even knew that the HD gene existed, let alone that their own dad had it.

Brian was the third of those four children, with two brothers and one sister. I remember his surviving sister, my auntie Joyce, who stepped in a lot to help him later in his life, telling us at his funeral that he had quite a temper as a teenager. I don't remember constant explosions of anger from my early years in the way that my younger sister Wendy does from her early years, so I think the Huntington's-induced anger came later. On the other hand, for the sake of even-handedness, I should say Wendy's feeling is that Dad was just better at covering it up in the earlier years of the marriage and that the tensions and aggression were always there.

There was that 'creative temperament' we referred to in his eulogy, with the story of the smashed typewriter. How much of that and of his teenage temper was down to his own passionate nature and how much might have been early signs of Huntington's I guess we will never know, despite my attempt to split this chapter into two neat halves, before HD and after HD. There is the stereotype of the fiery, hard-drinking, driven newsman, and that was definitely the culture of British journalism that Dad worked in. Judging by his clashes with people at work, it is one that he lived up to.

Anyway, back to his childhood. His father left home when he was very young, so Dad grew up without a dad of his own. It's partly because my grandfather left the family home and they virtually lost touch with him that they did not discover until much later that he died of Huntington's Disease, or Huntington's Chorea as it was called then.

Was it the Huntington's that made him act selfishly in leaving four young children with their mother to struggle along while he started a new life with a new woman? Who knows? Who can ever know? We know that Huntington's makes you act selfishly. But a lot of men have done the same thing without having an HD gene to blame.

Life was hard for a single mother with four children in the late 1930s and 1940s. But my grandma Lil (Elizabeth) worked hard to

keep the family from poverty. Dad got into grammar school where he had to put up with some teasing because the family could only afford a second-hand school uniform.

Starting a family of his own

He met my mum at Methodist Sunday school, aged 14, and they became teen sweethearts, marrying when they were 21. They had a happy marriage until the Huntington's began to change my father's behaviour.

My recollection of Dad from those years is confirmed by old journalist colleagues of his who remembered him fondly enough to come to his funeral decades later. He was a very intelligent and creative man, they told me when I asked what their memories of him were. He was good fun to be around and had a great sense of humour.

I also remember him being very supportive to me as a dad, always giving me advice if I needed it. My friends from school thought he and my mum were great, as they were always made welcome at our home. It was open house, virtually, for any waifs and strays among our schoolfriends. They preferred to come around to our house and be fed by my mum, then stay as long as possible, than to go home, because they liked the atmosphere in our house.

In fact, until Huntington's tore us apart I remember us being a very happy and close family. We went on picnics and family holidays, camping and touring across Europe. I think my mum has slightly different memories of the enormous long-haul trip Dad dragged us all on across Europe, since his thinking and planning may have been a little sketchy and chaotic by then. I get the impression in retrospect that it was left to my mum to manage the practical details of this great adventure, which involved three small children, including a baby, being driven across half a dozen countries, up mountains and down valleys.

I recall my dad being a great believer in the power of positive thinking. Having succeeded against the backdrop of a difficult childhood, he wanted us to know that if you believe in yourself you can achieve anything. It's not the problems and setbacks in life that are thrown at you, but the way you deal with them that counts, is what I picked up from him in those years. Now I know how valuable that attitude towards life is.

We lived in Whitley Bay, a small town outside Newcastle in Northumberland, on England's spectacular and often stormy north-east coast, until I was 12. My father worked for a TV programme called *Look North* in Newcastle. My mum looked after the three of us small kids. When he got a job in London, we moved down to a village called Ledwell in Oxfordshire. We began to see less of him from then on, as he travelled around for work quite a bit as well as working 80 miles away at the BBC's television headquarters in London. By now Dad was in his early thirties. Time, I guess, to take off the rose-coloured retrospective spectacles, and acknowledge the arrival on the scene of the effects of Huntington's.

After Huntington's began to take hold

It was a long way from the Brian I describe above to this:

It was Friday evening in our house in Chipping Norton, Oxfordshire. I was 23 and working in London, having left home five years previously to go to college. I had come home for the weekend for my best friend's wedding the next day. My dad had been drinking and was becoming increasingly abusive to my mum. She had confided in me in recent years that their marriage was becoming a nightmare for her and that he hit her. When I was a teenager I had heard it from my room at night. But Mum had spent years covering up for him and keeping the extent of his violence a secret from us children.

He was becoming increasingly abusive towards her that night, blaming her for all kinds of things that had gone wrong in his life. I

saw him raise his hand to her, the first time he'd done that in my presence. I now know that my brother and sister had seen this side of him more than once while I was living away. When my brother Geoff was at home from sea – he was an engineer in the merchant navy – he had on more than one occasion to pull my dad off my mum and warn him not to touch her.

On this occasion, to divert Dad's attention from Mum, I said, 'Don't hit her. Hit me!' I just assumed this would shame him into backing off, as he'd never hit me, not once in my entire life. To my shock, and my mum's, he came at me. I retreated out of the room into the hallway to escape his blows. He followed me, hitting me from behind. I fell under the telephone table in the hall and played dead. He walked away. I didn't go to the wedding the next day because I was covered in bruises. Although my mum had put up with being hit herself, this was the first time he had attacked one of her children. She started divorce proceedings almost immediately and left him as fast as she could.

Years of decline

Dad was 44 when the climactic incident mentioned above virtually ended his marriage to my mum. He had 15 more years to live. Looking back now, I can see that my mum had held things together, under increasing strain, over at least the previous decade, while Dad spiralled out of control. He lost a series of jobs, usually after spectacular rows with his bosses. His hitherto very successful career with the BBC had sputtered to an end.

Unable to find senior level work in television any more, we now think because he had developed a reputation as being unreliable and erratic, he had decided to go back to becoming a newspaper-man. He bought a local newspaper in Kent, south-east England, planning to run it as owner-editor. With Huntington's you tend to become the centre of your own universe, which may be why Dad's plans, to our surprise, included having the whole family work for

him. This family enterprise would include Geoff as advertising manager, me as a fellow journalist and Mum presumably doing everything else. Wendy was still too young to be roped in as unpaid labour. I suppose he would have had her making the tea.

I did write a couple of fashion columns for his paper. But my brother had his own career and my mum wisely refused to get involved. The paper limped along for a short while with Dad at its helm before crashing and burning financially. Dad was bust. In the process, Mum lost the large family house we used to have in Ledwell, and all financial security. That's how we had ended up in a much smaller home in the nearby town of Chipping Norton.

Mum had started working part-time years before. I didn't realize, at the time, that her relatively small income from this work was often what had put bread on the table. In that final decade and and a half or so of their marriage, Dad was increasingly away filming. I discovered later that if he was in a bad mood with Mum when he left on a trip, which often lasted a week or two or even more, he would leave her with no money. That explained the occasional family activity that I never quite understood at the time, when Mum would wrap us three kids up in hats, coats and scarves, and drag us out (with me complaining bitterly) to gather wood 'for fun'. It was in fact to heat the house as she had no money to pay the utility bills.

My mum still keeps much of what she had to put up with in those years to herself. But I know she had to put up with almost casual violence. As Huntington's makes your mood change suddenly, she can't have been able to predict it. One of the few occasions she told me about emphasized how the violence would come out of the blue. They were in the front room having an apparently normal conversation. Something had angered him, but there was no clue. He reached up to sweep the curtains closed with a movement of his arm and, as part of the same movement, swung around and punched her.

Looking back, I probably began to notice small changes in my dad's behaviour from when I was about 17. He had always been slightly eccentric, in that scatty, absent-minded way that creative people often are. So at first we may not have been aware that anything was wrong. He began to lose his temper with my sister over unimportant issues, which was unusual for him. He also seemed to become forgetful and began suffering from depression and twitching muscles. We thought that these symptoms may have been because he drank too much. He'd always been a bit of a boozer and it was part of the job in British journalism. In hindsight, he must have started developing the symptoms in his thirties, the same as me.

After the break-up

So, for years after his break-up with my mum, we hated him. There was continuing fear, too; my mum and younger sister Wendy, who was still a teenager at the time, were terrified of him. After they divorced, my mum made every effort to ensure he couldn't find out where they lived.

Dad had a job by this time editing a magazine in the Middle East, only returning to England two or three times a year. I agreed to see him once for lunch on one of these occasions. I was by this time with Phil and he, Bromley and I met Dad at a restaurant in the West End. Dad was with his boss. Something odd I noticed at the time but didn't register as significant was that a couple of times Dad's hand fluttered up into the air and down again for no apparent reason. His boss, with whom he had become friends, was sitting next to him. On one occasion he caught Dad's hand just as it started to move up from the table and pushed it back down again, looking with an annoyed expression at Dad. Dad glanced at him and glanced down slightly sheepishly. I got the impression this was something that had happened before.

Falling down

I discovered later that Dad's symptoms became more severe in the years he worked in Kuwait. One day while working on a project, he fell over and dropped his camera. He went to the doctor for an explanation for the stumbling and clumsiness, but they focused on something else. They discovered that he had a localized form of skin cancer because of spending so much time in the Middle-Eastern sun over the previous couple of years. Consequently his problems with balance and the resulting fall were forgotten.

He came home to England to have the skin cancer treated. They removed a cancerous mole from his face and that was the end of that problem. The job in Kuwait also ended. I don't know why but I guess the quality of his work had slipped. My grandma Lil died around this time. Dad apparently decided to return to his roots. He bought her flat in Newcastle, lived and worked from it, trying to make a living first on local newspapers and then as a freelance journalist. He was increasingly stretched financially and by this time had real trouble walking. He ended up with the occasional job such as writing a regular column for a local paper that each week looked at the historical origins of a different local family surname. A far cry from his time as a senior producer and editor at the BBC.

We all had very little to do with Dad over these years. It was while he was living up in the north-east of England and trying to find a reason for his increasing physical disability that he was diagnosed with cerebellar ataxia. Sadly this was a misdiagnosis. Cerebellar ataxia is also a progressive disease that comes on later in life, but it affects people physically and not mentally or emotionally as Huntington's does. It is an awful illness to be sure, but cerebellar ataxia carries with it far fewer whammies than Huntington's.

Dad comes to London

Out of the blue, I received a letter from Dad saying he was moving to London, where I lived at the time, and wanted a reconciliation. I decided to give him a chance. It turned out he had somehow swapped his mum's flat for a supported flat in central London. It was part of a cluster of flats for elderly and disabled people that had a support worker on call and alarm cords in the flat that the resident could pull for assistance if they fell.

As I got re-acquainted with him over the occasional lunch, cup of coffee and so on, it became clear something was seriously wrong with him. His walking was wobbly. His thinking seemed eccentric. He had hatched a plan recently to buy land in Bolivia and farm it. He had even gone out there to look at the land he was planning to buy. There wasn't even a road leading to it, just a dirt track. It was a patch of jungle. Luckily, Dad didn't go ahead with it. I assume he used that money to buy his mum's flat instead, as it was all he had left.

Dad had a word processor in his flat and he spent a lot of time writing off letters asking for work with newspapers and the BBC. He became increasingly frustrated at the lack of response. Throughout this time, I discovered later, he was being financially supported by his sister Joyce. He was never again successful in finding a job.

I remember being out in the car with him and Phil in central London, Dad sitting in the front seat next to Phil, who was driving, and me in the back. We had a little two-door car and Dad couldn't get into the back. We were taking him to lunch. We drove past the offices in Holborn of the *Daily Mirror*, one of Britain's biggest tabloid newspapers at the time. 'I almost bought that last month, but bloody Barclays wouldn't lend me the money,' he said. 'Pardon? You bought the *Daily Mirror*?' I said from the back, not having heard him properly over the traffic. I thought he was saying that he'd bought a copy of the newspaper that morning and was about to tell us a story he had read in it. The conversation moved on to

something else. Months later, when clearing out his flat, we found an angry letter from him to Barclays Bank berating them for refusing even to answer the letter he had sent them asking for several million pounds to buy the *Daily Mirror*, which he had been planning to edit himself.

During this period of his life, Dad joined and left all the major political parties in the country. He had been a member of the Liberal Democrats for years. Yet one day when I went to his flat he had Conservative leaflets all over the place, told me he had joined them and they had the answer to all the country's problems. Next time I saw him he had Labour leaflets all over the flat and spent ages criticizing the Conservatives and telling me why he was now a Labour activist. When I saw him again a few months later he had joined the Green Party.

Discovering it's Huntington's Disease

A few months later – I was 34 by then – Dad wrote to tell me his sister had tracked down their father's death certificate and cause of death was given as Huntington's Disease. None of his family had known. Suddenly everything was clear. My dad had inherited it. As we looked into it and found out more about the disease, we realized that there was finally an explanation for his strange behaviour and violence.

His increasingly odd behaviour went on for several more years until he was finally admitted to a mental hospital in London, having tried to commit suicide by taking an overdose of paracetamol. We found a nursing home in the Forest of Dean in Gloucestershire that could take him. The patients there were mostly elderly people and he was only in his fifties. There were two other people there with Huntington's, one a bit younger than my dad, one older. The staff there were brilliant. While he was in the nursing home we tried to move on from the negative way we had perceived him, and to see him and his past differently. But it was a terrible strain on everybody.

We realized at one level that all along he had been very ill. But that didn't cancel out the pain that had been inflicted on everyone. I visited him as often as I could, though it was quite a long way to travel with two young sons. The radio in his room was always on when we visited. It was tuned permanently to BBC Radio 4, the news and current affairs station. He may not have been able to work for the BBC he loved any more, but he remained attached to them and to his newsman past by the umbilical cord of the BBC's news output. I think he was pleased to see us. He was in a wheelchair by then occasionally, and sometimes walking with a frame. He could still talk but it was quite hard to understand him.

After two years in the home he died, aged 59. In those final two years in the home at least he was reconciled with his children and met his grandchildren, whom he'd been estranged from for years. Phil and I went to clear out his belongings from his room, one of the most painful things I've ever done. As we passed his nicotine-stained things out through the window, all wrapped up in black plastic bags, a male nurse walked into Dad's old room and began helping us.

He said: 'I just wanted to say I got to know your dad and really liked him. We had a lot of enjoyable chats sitting out in the grounds in the sun. He was a clever and interesting person to listen to.

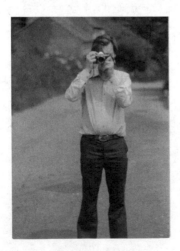

Always had his radio on. Always knew what was going on in the world and could talk about anything. I know you all had your troubles, but I could tell he was a nice man and he loved all of you. It's a terrible shame.' He was. And it is. I'm so glad that even at that stage of his life, after 30 years of the illness covering up the real Brian like ivy growing over a wall, someone was astute and caring enough to glimpse him as he really was, behind the Huntington's. I'm so glad to know that he was still there.

CHAPTER 8

Tips for Living with Huntington's Disease

Both my husband Phil and older son Brom read a lot of self-improvement books to help them become stronger in dealing with HD. So, I asked Phil to put this chapter together...

Making yourself stronger

Here are a few ideas for how to gain and maintain the strength you need to deal with HD. Different members of our family have used all of these tips and will continue to do so. We're talking months and years here for this to take effect, but HD moves slowly, so you can keep pace or keep ahead of it.

Dump the emotional baggage

We all carry emotional baggage around with us. I mean the insecurities and self-doubt that lie under the surface. Within us, often subconsciously, are the fears that developed from unhappy experiences, the sense of our own limitations that became set in concrete every time we failed or were told we had failed, or every time we got hurt.

To become stronger so you can deal with Huntington's, you may want to deal with these inner demons. It's like cleaning a house. If you don't get them tidied up and put away in their boxes, they will be a constant distraction, tugging on your coat tails and sapping your energy. If you fail to deal with them, you'll be quicker to anger, less confident and have less of a buffer of calm to draw on. And you'll be more tired. Some of the steps below can help.

Talk yourself stronger

…with family, selected friends, counsellor, shrink, doctor, other people with experience of HD, support workers, other carers or people at risk. HD can seem so big that you feel powerless to talk about it without sinking into depression or anger. Not talking about it lets all your fears about it stay unformed and scary, like a knot in your stomach. Have the occasional rant to selected friends: you will soon know which one or two can deal with it and which can't. Counsellors can be a great source of techniques for rethinking things, steering your thoughts away from negative 'I can't do this!' paralysis. So can friends and family. Talk to other carers about what they do if you are a carer.

Don't go it alone

This is really part of 'talk yourself strong'. Ask for help and advice. It's often the small problems that are *so* frustrating. People come up with brilliant ideas to solve them. We were having increasing trouble getting Sandy's contact lenses in once a month and discarding the old ones. She could no longer do it herself. I took over, but after a few months I couldn't do it either. We got to the stage where she had only one lens in for a couple of weeks, giving her a cock-eyed view of life, and headaches. I was getting desperate. She didn't seem bothered!

Sandy's mum said, 'I've been thinking about your problem: if she lies on her back with her head on a pillow, her head can't move as much.' It was a stroke of genius and worked immediately. Instead of 20 increasingly frustrating minutes of Sandy sitting on the edge of the bath or standing in front of the bathroom mirror, with me reaching around to her eye from behind and dropping the lens endlessly, it was in her eye in seconds. A daft example, maybe, but a sound principle: constantly ask other people for ideas on how to solve all the small problems that HD throws up every day.

Vent

I have two or three friends who constantly want to know how I am. I mean *really* know. They are the ones who don't accept 'Fine, thanks,' but keep digging. One phones every now and again 'just in case you need a moan'. Another wants to know in great detail what little things I struggle with sometimes with the HD and she is then astonishingly creative and generous in coming up with a stream of possible solutions, all of which seem brilliant and many of which work.

When you are too befuddled with it all, having a fresh and willing brain like that to help you out is the greatest gift friends can give. You will soon find there are one, maybe two, or if you are supremely lucky, three friends who can and want to operate at that level with you.

Others may just want to help by taking you away from HD and getting you drunk or otherwise showing you a good time. Which is great. And others won't know how to cope with it and may not contact you at all. They're just not sure what to do. You need times when you don't talk about HD at all so you can forget it for a while. Call up a friend and suggest going out, with one condition – that you *don't* talk about HD. They'll probably be as relieved as you.

If you've neglected your friends and maybe lost some you value along the way, as I have, then get back in touch and explain that you

lost the plot for a bit as you tried to come to terms with HD. I can't stress enough: don't go it alone. As my brilliant counsellor keeps saying to me, 'Who do you think you are: Superman?'

Read yourself stronger

There are a lot of books out there about making yourself stronger, if you are the reading type. And, as you are reading this, that suggests you might be. Here are a couple:

The Other 90%: How to Unlock Your Vast, Untapped Potential for Leadership & Life by Robert Cooper (2001)

I love this book. I find it constantly uplifting and inspirational. It's full of reminders like 'Remember the funniest thing that happened today… In one study of 50 married couples, psychologists found that humor accounted for 70 percent of the difference in happiness between couples who enjoyed life and those who didn't' (p.131). Some of the things that happen with HD can be extremely funny. Learn to laugh at them and look for non-HD things that keep you laughing, too. Laughter breaks you free. It helps you, says the author, 'slow down and take a good look, shaking free of the mindset of exhaustion, and reclaiming more of your life'.

The 7 Habits of Highly Effective People by Stephen Covey (1989)

You don't have to read all of it. And the author, Stephen Covey, isn't for everyone. But, one thing particularly useful in it is his point about how we react when criticized or attacked; how we don't realize that we are programmed to react angrily and defensively or to withdraw into ourselves, from childhood. But, in fact, when you are suddenly attacked there is a space in which you can choose how to react. HD leads to outbursts. You know this if you live with someone with HD. The suddenness of the verbal assault – if you're

lucky, it's verbal – can knock you sideways emotionally as it comes out of the blue.

You don't have to go with the programming and react defensively, aggressively or feel belittled and knocked down. You can choose how to react. I still have the occasional moment, particularly when I'm tired, of responding with 'Well, if I'm that stupid, then make your own dinner next time,' when I know Sandy can't. But that's usually down to tiredness (see 'sleep yourself strong', below).

The Tao of Pooh and the Te of Piglet by Benjamin Hoff (2002)
See Dr Hin's advice, below.

Laugh yourself stronger

Just to reinforce that point from Robert K. Cooper's book, above: 'Don't be afraid to laugh at yourself and even at HD. It's probably the best known treatment for HD at this time' (Paulsen 1999, p.21).

Sleep yourself stronger

Don't be tempted to stay up after everyone is finally in bed to clear up and do all the stuff you couldn't get done when they were awake. I know. I've tried it.

Similarly, be wary of slipping into using the night-time as your own time to stay awake and recover with a few hours of no one making demands on you. A friend of mine is the main carer in an HD family and I swap experiences with her. She said this, which I immediately identified with:

> When they are all in bed, that's my time. So, instead of going to sleep myself, I read, wind down, watch DVDs, sort through in my head all that happened during the day, plan the next day. It's as if I feel unable to relax during the day because there is a constant call on my time. But then I don't get to bed till 3 am and am exhausted next morning.

Couples where one person has HD will commonly get to the stage where the person with HD moves around so much at night that the other person gets no sleep. Sleeping pills, if the doctor thinks it's appropriate, do help the person with HD to have a less disturbed sleep. But the partner often will still need to find other sleeping arrangements to avoid being kicked and pushed out of bed by the sleeping partner throughout the night. This can lead to an ongoing row, as sleeping separately can be seen as a symbolic end to a marriage. We went through this row. It lasted months. I now sleep in a spare bed in the basement. We both sleep better for it.

Long-term sleep deprivation will bring you down and make you less able to cope. If you have HD, lack of sleep will make you irritable and easily angered. Guard your sleep jealously. Looking after yourself is vital if you are to be strong enough to help look after others.

What about you?

For carers in particular, set aside regular time for yourself and don't lose track of your friends and pastimes or hobbies. Maybe you have to do less of them. But don't lose them completely. Or you lose yourself. I've done that. The trick here is don't fall into the trap of making yourself indispensable – or assuming you are indispensable. Demand and take any help social services, other family members, doctors, voluntary agencies, neighbours (well, ask, don't demand, in their case), whoever can give.

For the person with HD, if your past interests and hobbies become undoable, you and the people who support you need to try new ones till you find something you like, or variations on the old ones. If you used to play football, but can't now, maybe you want to go and watch games regularly instead. That's just an example. It's easy for support people – family and care workers – to focus on immediate needs like food, cleaning and the like. Don't let them forget that your life needs some fun and recreation, too.

Dr Hin's tips

Dr Hin, one of our family doctors, talked me through how to use some of the world's major religions or belief systems to reframe how you deal with Huntington's Disease. It was very wise advice. Here's a potted version of the three he used as examples. Any errors of interpretation are mine. You don't have to follow these religions, of course, just use the useful parts of them to help rethink Huntington's and how you deal with it.

Buddhism

Useful for reinterpreting suffering as what life is about: instead of a terrible thing you have been landed with, it provides an opportunity for growth. If you can't get away from it (suffering) then use it to grow stronger.

Tao-ism

Useful for acceptance. Tao-ism is all about going with the flow. Dr Hin recommends Benjamin Hoff's *The Tao of Pooh* (see 'Read yourself strong' above). He even wears Winnie The Pooh ties as a reminder. Nice touch. I've read other Tao-inspired books. It's particularly useful for keeping calm and avoiding arguments.

Confucianism

This is all about control and order. Confucius said the calm that order creates starts within the family and flows outwards. This is a useful way of thinking to help counter the daily chaos and unpredictability that HD can bring to the family home. People with HD often feel far more comfortable and less stressed with an ordered routine to the day, so they know what to expect next. Carers, similarly, find that HD pulls you in the direction of chaos all the time, so establishing as much of an orderly environment and routine as possible helps prevent the feeling that life is spinning out of control.

'The profound impact of disordered behaviour on families is at last being recognized by professionals' (Snowdon 2001).

Hope or Faith?

People in long-term difficult situations often refer to Hope (often, as I typed it here, with a capital letter at the front) as being their greatest source of strength. I used to think so too; that Hope was the strongest attribute you could have in a sea of troubles. It made sense that Hope was the treasure to fly out last of all from Pandora's mythical box and give humanity the strength to deal with all the horrors that had poured out before it.

Years ago, I saw a wonderful example of belief in Hope, and the image has stayed with me for over a decade. Odd then, that my advice now should be to abandon all hope when faced with a long-term difficult situation, and cultivate something else instead, something far more powerful. I'll get on to that in a minute. First, the example of Hope in action I saw years ago that touched me so much at the time.

The story of Hope

We used to live near an overland section of the Tube (the London Underground) that runs above and alongside a playground. When Danny was a baby he would react ecstatically every time he saw a train coming on this raised section of track, kicking his legs, waving his arms and laughing unstoppably as it went by. Only babies seem capable of being consumed with such total delight and it was a wonderful thing to see.

I used to sit him on a swing in the playground, with a perfect view upwards to the train track running along the viaduct above, and we'd wait, and he'd peer into the distance. Every couple of minutes Dan would hear one coming, shout, 'Train! Train!' and point. I'd sit on the bench next to him reading a book. He would

happily sit there for hours if you let him, a rapt train-spotter at just 18 months.

One Sunday afternoon we were sitting there waiting for the next train. I glanced up at the slide a few yards over from the swings. A little girl, about four years old maybe, was standing at the bottom step of the slide, her hand on one rail, looking up to the top. Her mum was standing to one side, watching her. The little girl had callipers on her legs and very thick-lensed, large glasses. She looked frail. She glanced at her mum. 'You can do it,' her mum said quietly.

The little girl managed to get one leg up onto the bottom rung, then swing her other leg up to the next step. She was having to hang on tight as her legs weren't strong enough to balance her, and she was swaying a little on the callipers. Halfway up, she looked over at her mother anxiously. Her mum pushed her hands further down into her pockets and didn't move. That must have taken a great effort of will. She was, purposely I'm sure, just a bit too far away to catch the girl if she fell. And both of them knew it. The ground surface was rubber but even so, it looked a long way to drop. 'You can do it,' the mother said quietly again.

The little girl struggled to the top, sat down with a clunk and beamed over at her mum, who came close, reached up and stroked her hand. 'Well done, Hope. I knew you could do it,' she said.

When I heard her name, I pictured (quite possibly wrongly, but it struck me as likely) this little girl being born four years earlier, maybe prematurely, with weak limbs, poor eyesight and a tough future. Perhaps it was even touch and go whether she would survive. But she had. And her parents decided to give her the name Hope as she stepped out into an unforgiving world on wobbly legs, peering at it through thick glasses. Her name, I assumed, was chosen as a kind of shield, a reminder of what she had to develop in herself to overcome the obstacles she would face. Obstacles like an apparently unclimbable slide for a little girl in callipers. She would have to become Hope incarnate.

For ten years I used the mental image of the little girl struggling up the slide as a kind of reinforcement every time Huntington's Disease threw something tough at us. 'If a little girl can push on with Hope against what seemed an insurmountable obstacle, then so can we,' was the reinforcing mechanism I called on in my head.

But, a year or so ago I realized I had got it completely wrong. It wasn't the power of Hope her mother was exposing her to, proving it was strong enough to get her up that slide. It was the power of Faith: 'I *knew* you could do it, Hope.' Faith was the lesson the mother was passing on. 'You can do this insurmountable thing, and realizing that you can do it will help give you the faith to face the next scary thing in your life, and the next, and the next. Because, each time, you will know you are capable of far more than you think you are.' That's what she was teaching her daughter.

Hope carries within it the possibility of failure. It has a seed of doubt lodged in its middle. If you hope you are strong enough, you are admitting the possibility that you won't be. Faith just knows you can triumph over whatever you face and not go under, if you just maintain the will to go on. There is a powerful calm and sense of strength that comes with that. Compared with Faith, Hope is a wimp.

Faith in what?

Well, if you're religious, you don't need that question asked. I'm not, so the answer was harder to reach for me. In fact, it took years. In a sense, it doesn't matter what you find Faith in, as long as you find it. There's a Joss Whedon sci-fi movie, *Serenity*. A preacher in the film tells the hero that he will only prevail against the evil empire if he believes. 'Sorry, I'm not religious,' says the hero. 'You don't have to believe what I believe. Just believe in something. They believe in their cause. You won't stop them unless you believe in yours,' says the preacher. Or something like that. I'm paraphrasing.

Where does strength come from? From belief, from conviction of some kind. I've always believed people are capable of far more than they are called on to give. I used to be fascinated by those occasional stories of people finding hidden strength when they needed it – mothers caught in a car crash who lift a car to rescue their child trapped under it, that kind of thing. Many, possibly all, of those stories are urban myths, of course. There's a half-remembered quote in my head that goes something like, 'If you look at what people are capable of compared with what they achieve, life is endlessly disappointing.' Well, Huntington's gives you an extraordinary opportunity to raise your game. To draw on another quote, what doesn't kill you makes you stronger.

I know that sounds glib, and I know you may be thinking, 'Yes, but for the person with HD, it *does* kill you, and if you are at risk, it *might* kill you.' The triumph over the illness comes in making the absolute most of every second that you and they have; of wringing every positive thing you can out of their and your life. And that is a lesson that applies to all of us, whether we have HD in the family or not.

Ordinary people

Ordinary people are capable of absolute acts of heroism, and can find extraordinary strength, particularly in situations where someone you care for is under attack. In the school playground I wasn't much of a fighter. But a couple of times, when I spotted my cousin Barry being bullied or outnumbered in a playground showdown, I turned into a fearless avenger and charged in with no thought of 'Uh-oh, I can't do this.' Barry did the same for me frequently. You'll be familiar with that feeling, maybe from your dim and distant past, I'm sure. Get in touch with it again. Remember a time when you were brave on behalf of someone else, not so much fearless as overcoming the fear. Picture it over and over again in your head. It's a useful source of strength.

OK, I've just heard this on the radio from a monk, and it helps reconcile the God/no God thing. Here's what he said: 'God has no hands. God has no feet. God has no mouth except ours. It's up to us.' I love that.

So, believe in God if you like, but don't look outside for his or her intervention. This one's up to you. There's that powerful Quaker belief that 'there is that of God in each of us', which makes the same point the monk was making. Or don't believe in God if you like. But *do* believe in yourself and each other. There is a vast untapped source of strength in our family and over the past couple of years I have developed faith that we will be OK whatever happens, just by watching them deal with the challenges they face. Like watching Hope get to the top of that slide.

Appendix: Useful Resources

There is a lot of information out there. The problem is being over-whelmed by it. So, this is just a short selection that we recommend.

'I have HD' sheet

Carol Dutton, the Regional Care Advisor who covers our area for the UK Huntington's Disease Association, helped put together an A4 sheet that is a brilliant 60-second crash course to get people inside the head of someone with HD. It's a useful reminder for family members, friends and informal carers as well as a great introduction for professionals such as new staff at a care home who may need to be brought up to speed quickly as a prelude to finding out more about it through proper training. It reads like this...

I have HD. This means:

- I like my routine.
- I do *one* thing at a time.
- You need to get my attention and then tell me what you want.
- Give me time to answer. Don't repeat what you said or put it another way; this makes it difficult for me to answer.
- Listen to what I say – it takes a lot of effort.
- I don't know how to *wait*! If I need something I need it *now*.
- I need a constant supply of little snacks and drinks.
- My brain gets stuck on thinking about important things, so I repeat the same words a lot.
- There is only one solution to a problem/question.
- I remember my life before I came here.

- Sometimes I'm scared of the future – I think a lot.

- I can still enjoy things and have fun.

- I used to be independent, had a normal life, and make my own decisions. I don't want to change more than I have to.

A brilliant book

Huntington's and Me: A Guide for Young People by Alison Gray (2000)

This is the best written resource we have ever found on Huntington's Disease. It is *so* easy to understand and so clearly written that we recommend it for anyone, not just young people.

It explains in simple and clear language all sorts of technical issues that we had struggled with including, for example, the implications of the different possible numbers of CAG repeats on chromosome 4 and how that can affect people differently, which we had read about elsewhere but just couldn't get our heads around properly. Plus beautifully written insights and advice from young people themselves and from Alison Gray, the author.

It can be obtained through the UK Huntington's Disease Association, www.hda.org.uk, email info@hda.org.uk.

A guide for doctors

A Physician's Guide to the Management of Huntington's Disease: Pharmacological and Non-Pharmacological Interventions by Adam Rosenblatt *et al.* (1999)

With the honourable exception of our own brilliant family doctors, especially Dr Cornwall, who is my main doctor, families with Huntington's report that their family doctors commonly lack the knowledge to provide the support the family needs.

If your family falls into this category, invest in this guide for your family doctor and give it to him/her. Better, persuade them to buy it themselves. If you are a doctor yourself or a professional who works with this illness and you know of doctors who need to be betterinformed, point them at this guide.

It also includes useful coping strategies for family members such as 'for instance, an HD-affected person should turn off radios, television, and telephones, and limit conversations while cooking dinner' because divided attention becomes difficult.

We got our doctor a copy from the UK Huntington's Disease Association.

Understanding behaviour (or 'behavior' if you are in the US)

Two very good reports that are a great help in making sense of Huntington's and are both full of insights and tips on, for example, avoiding conflict can be found on the web as Microsoft Word document downloads by searching the titles and author names with Google. That's how we found them. They were on several websites last time we looked:

Understanding Challenging Behavior in Huntington's Disease by Julie Snowden (2001)
This is about 12 A4 pages long, and full of useful insights such as:

> ...problem behaviors are most likely to occur in the home and to be directed towards those family members and care-givers to whom the person with HD is closest, not towards relative strangers. Thus, behavioral problems are likely to be underestimated by outsiders. (p.1)

> One common characteristic is that people with HD may seem content to do nothing. If left to their own devices, they might lie in bed all day or sit watching television. This can of course, be exasperating to a busy partner, who may resent the fact that all duties and responsibilities fall on them. However, the person with HD is not being lazy. The brain changes in HD mean that there is a loss of drive and initiative, so that the person cannot self-motivate. The stimulus needs to come from outside rather than within. Doing tasks together can be helpful since the activities of the partner acts as a stimulus to the person with HD. (p.3)

Understanding Behaviour in Huntington's Disease: A Practical Guide
for Individuals, Families, and Professionals Coping with HD **by Jane**
Paulsen (1999)
This report is about 50 A4 pages long, and includes more technical detail
than Julie Snowden's report, but is still full of useful stuff for the
layperson like us, for example:

> Since the caudate [part of the brain] is unable to regulate
> properly (in other words, the gate needs oil), people with HD
> need a regulated environment that provides daily structure
> and routine upon which they can depend.
>
> Because the caudate cannot get the information from the
> frontal lobes to decide what is the most important thing to do
> next or how to order the day's activities, a person with HD
> relies on external sources to structure the day and make
> decisions.
>
> ...A particularly important time to minimize distractions
> to diminish circuit overload is during mealtime. Swallowing
> difficulties due to impaired muscle control and functioning
> create the need for concentration when eating meals. Distrac-
> tions while eating can increase the chances of choking and
> inhaling food or liquid into the lungs. (p.7)

Websites and leaflets

The Huntington's associations in various countries provide useful information, advice and updates on latest research on their websites and in
leaflets (often downloadable from the websites).

Australian Huntington's Disease Association
www.huntingtonsaustralia.asn.au

Huntington Society of Canada
www.hsc-ca.org

Huntington's Disease Assocation UK
www.hda.org.uk

Huntington's Disease Society of America
www.hdsa.org

International Huntington Association
www.huntington-assoc.com

Huntington's Disease Associations New Zealand
Huntington's Disease Association (Auckland) Inc
Email: huntingtonsakld@xtra.co.nz

Huntington's Disease Association (Wellington) Inc
Email: info.wellingtonhda@xtra.co.nz

References

Cooper, Robert K. (2001) *The Other 90%: How to Unlock Your Vast, Untapped Potential for Leadership and Life.* New York: Crown Business.

Covey, Stephen (1989) *The 7 Habits of Highly Effective People.* London: Simon & Schuster.

Gray, Alison (2000) *Huntington's and Me: A Guide for Young People.* Wellington: Huntington's Disease Association.

Hoff, Benjamin (2002) *The Tao of Pooh and the Te of Piglet.* London: Egmont.

Kressly, Esther Neufeld (1995) 'A Love Story.' Chicago, IL. University of Chicago Library. Available at: www.lib.uchicago.edu (accessed 10 July 2006).

Paulsen, Jane S. (1999) *Understanding Behaviour in Huntington's Disease: A Practical Guide for Individuals, Families, and Professionals Coping with HD.* Ontario: Huntington Society of Canada. Available from http://huntingtondisease.tripod.com/understandingbehaviour (accessed 26 July 2006).

Rosenblatt, Adam, Ranen, Neal G., Nance, Martha A. and Paulsen, Jane S. (1999) *A Physician's Guide to the Management of Huntington's Disease: Pharmacological and Non-Pharmacological Interventions.* New York: Huntington's Disease Society of America (reprinted in the UK with permission by the Huntington's Disease Association, London, 2002).

Snowden, Julie (2001) *Understanding Challenging Behaviour in Huntington's Disease.* Paper presented at the 14th International Meeting of the International Huntington Association held in Denmark. The Netherlands: International Huntington Association. Available at http://huntingtondisease.tripod.com/understandingbehaviorotherresources/id2.html (accessed 15 July 2006).